Soy!
Soy!
Soy!

Soy! Soy! Soy!

Enjoy Soyfoods' Benefits in Delicious Recipes

Jeanette Parsons Egan

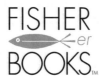

FISHER
BOOKS™

Publishers: Howard W. Fisher, Helen V. Fisher

Managing Editor: Sarah Trotta

Editor: Helen V. Fisher

Production & Interior design: Randy Schultz

Photography: ©1999 Lois Ellen Frank, LOIS Photography

Food styling: Jeanette Parsons Egan

Cover images: ©1998 Adobe Systems Incorporated Digit Art Clip Art on CD-ROM

Cover design: Randy Schultz

Index: Michelle B. Graye

Published by Fisher Books, LLC
5225 W. Massingale Road
Tucson, Arizona 85743-8416
Tel: (520) 744-6110

Library of Congress Cataloging-in-Publication Data

Egan, Jeanette Parsons.
  Soy! soy! soy! : enjoy soyfoods' benefits in delicious recipes / Jeanette Parsons Egan.
    p. cm.
  ISBN 1-55561-174-5
  1. Cookery (Soybeans) 2. Soyfoods. I. Title.

TX803.S6 E34 1999
641.6'5655—dc21   99-040084
                                CIP

Notice: The information in this book is true and complete to the best of our knowledge. It is offered with no guarantees on the part of the author or Fisher Books. Author and publisher disclaim all liability in connection with use of this book.

Printed in U.S.A.
10 9 8 7 6 5 4 3 2 1

Nutrient analysis was calculated using The Food Processor® for Windows software program, version 6.0, copyright 1987-1995 by ESHA Research. Analysis does not include optional ingredients or variations. Where an ingredient amount is given as a range, the higher number is used for calculation purposes. The following abbreviations are used:

Cal = Calories
Prot = Protein
Carb = Carbohydrates
Fib = Fiber
Fat = Total fat
Chol = Cholesterol

Contents

Why I Love Soyfoods
vii

A Soyfoods Glossary
xxii

Appetizers
1

Soups
15

Salads
31

Main Dishes
49

Side Dishes
77

Breads
91

Breakfast Dishes
105

Desserts
127

Mail-Order Sources
153

Other Sources
154

Index
155

Dedication

To my husband, John, who tasted every recipe, made helpful suggestions and made the project fun. He is now a firm believer in "going soy."

Acknowledgments

Special thanks to Lorraine Freyer, who quickly lost her skepticism, for help with recipe testing. Thanks to all those tasters who ate the dishes, usually without knowing they contained soy.

Thanks to all those at Fisher Books who have been involved in this project, especially Sarah Trotta and Helen Fisher, and the late Bill Fisher, who first suggested that I do this book.

Why I Love Soyfoods

It seems as if every day more information is published about soyfoods and their health benefits. If you haven't already discovered *soyfoods*, the general term for all the different products made from soybeans, now is the perfect time to jump in! It's as easy as exploring your nearest supermarket, where you will find many new soy-based products, including several nonfat or low-fat options. According to one source, more than 200 new soy products are introduced to consumers each year.

Soyfoods are no longer just for vegetarians—they are for everyone. I consider soyfoods such as tofu, soybeans and soy beverages as much a part of my regular diet as fruits, vegetables, meats, dairy products and grains. Nor are they reserved only for recipes that fall into the "health" category. I include them in many of my dips, creamy soups, main-dish salads, hearty sandwiches and yummy desserts, from pie to "ice cream." I regularly serve them to guests!

For guests who haven't yet embraced the "soy revolution," I usually don't announce that the luscious dip or dessert I'm serving contains soy. I wait until someone says, "This is delicious! How did you make it?" Then I casually mention that in addition to the herbs, spices and other ingredients, the dish contains tofu or another soyfood. The usual response is, "But it's so good . . . it doesn't *taste* like tofu."

For those who believe that tofu is served only as "those white cubes," this requires a whole new way of thinking about soyfoods, particularly tofu. So far, no one I know has simply stopped eating just because they discovered the dish contained a soyfood! Instead, I hear lots of questions about my reasons for adding soyfoods when I cook. (More about this later. See *Why Eat Soyfoods?,* page viii.)

I consider soyfoods such as tofu, soybeans and soy beverages as much a part of my regular diet as fruits, vegetables, meats, dairy products and grains.

"But it's so good . . . it doesn't *taste* like tofu."

When I serve soyfoods, I usually find my guests are somewhat familiar with soy products and their health benefits. They either already use them or are eager to learn how to incorporate them into meals.

It's easy to cook with soyfoods, because they are no longer available only at natural-food stores or Asian markets. They are now stocked in major supermarkets across the country. Look for soyfoods in the produce section and in the refrigerated and frozen-food cases. Some products, such as canned soybeans, soynut butter and shelf-stable soy beverages, are found on grocery shelves.

Look for soyfoods in the produce section and in the refrigerated and frozen-food cases. Some products . . . are found on grocery shelves.

Why Eat Soyfoods?

Two important reasons health-conscious people are excited about eating soyfoods are that soy is good for us, and it is easily added to a normal diet. Soyfoods contain high-quality protein, fiber, lecithin and omega-three fatty acids in addition to nutrients such as folacin and other B vitamins, vitamin E, calcium, zinc and iron. All of these substances have nutritional value. In addition, soyfoods contain beneficial substances called *isoflavones*. (See box on opposite page.)

Soy's Health Benefits

There is much we *don't* know about the process by which soyfoods benefit human health. In some cases, isoflavones appear to combine with soy protein—and possibly other chemicals found in the soybean—to achieve certain beneficial effects. In other cases, the soy protein or an isoflavone alone seem to be enough to confer a health benefit.

Scientists still have much research to do before they understand everything about the complex interactions of the substances found in soyfoods. Until we know more, *get the benefits by eating soyfoods instead of taking an isoflavone supplement.* A supplement alone may not provide all the elements needed to confer the isoflavone's intended health benefit.

Researchers are studying at least four major medical conditions for which soy may be beneficial. These are heart disease, cancer, osteoporosis and menopause.

Isoflavones—Rich in Soyfoods

What are isoflavones and why should we eat them? These substances are just one of a group of compounds called phytochemicals *or plant* chemicals. *These compounds are not considered nutrients but they do affect the way the body functions. Soybeans are one of the richest sources of two isoflavones,* genistein *and* daidzein.

Reduces Heart Disease

Coronary heart disease is the major cause of death in the United States and Canada. Fighting coronary heart disease through one's diet can be effective, and soyfoods can help.

Lowers "bad" cholesterol. One of the best-researched and documented benefits of soy protein is its serum-lipid-lowering effect. Soy protein reduces the *LDL* or "bad" cholesterol levels in the bloodstream without reducing the *HDL* or "good" cholesterol levels. HDL levels may actually *increase* slightly. Individuals with extremely high cholesterol levels see the greatest reductions when they add soyfoods to their diet, but eating soy protein reduces LDL cholesterol levels even in those persons with normal cholesterol levels.

Serum triglycerides, another fat that at high levels is correlated with coronary heart disease, are also reduced. How soy protein exerts its influence on serum lipids is not fully understood. It is probably the result of a combination of factors.

May inhibit clot formation and arterial-plaque formation. The isoflavone genistein may inhibit clot formation and the growth of plaques in the artery walls. Clots and arterial plaques can cause heart attack or stroke. The beneficial action of genistein may be related to its role as an antioxidant in preventing the attack on LDL cholesterol by *free radicals* (unstable oxygen molecules). When LDL cholesterol is oxidized by free radicals, it accumulates in, and blocks, blood vessels.

Adds fiber to diet. Some soyfoods contain fiber. Fiber, particularly insoluble fiber, also helps reduce cholesterol by binding cholesterol and preventing its absorption from the intestinal tract. Soluble fiber is also important in controlling blood sugar levels in diabetics. Diabetes, particularly if uncontrolled, is another risk factor for heart disease. Whole soybeans, tempeh and soynuts are good sources of fiber.

Contains other nutrients for heart health. Other nutrients in soy that are related to heart health are folate and vitamin E. Folate is important in the metabolism of *homocysteine*, an amino acid normally found in the blood, and prevents its accumulation in the blood. High levels of homocysteine have been recently implicated as a risk factor for heart disease. Most of the vitamin E found in soy oil is removed and sold as supplements, but the remaining small amount is enough to be nutritionally significant. Vitamin E is an important antioxidant and reduces clot formation.

Helps Prevent Cancer

The fact that soyfoods are a diet staple in Asian countries is often cited to explain differences in the rates of prostate cancer, breast cancer and colon cancer between Asian and Western societies. Soybeans contain several chemicals that have anticancer properties. They include isoflavones, saponins, phytates, protease inhibitors and phytosterols. (Except for the isoflavones genistein and daidzein, these chemicals are found in other foods also.) The actions of these chemicals vary, from controlling cell growth and protecting cells from damage to inhibiting formation of new blood vessels that feed tumors. Other beneficial mechanisms may be involved also that are still unknown.

While the concentration in soyfoods varies, tofu, soy milk, tempeh, soy flour, textured soy protein and miso are rich sources of isoflavones.

Doctors are studying the effects of a high-soy diet in preventing and inhibiting growth of cancers of the skin, colon, prostate and breast. Most of the recent research has been done on the isoflavones in the area of hormone-dependent cancers, such as breast and prostate cancer. Laboratory studies with mice and rats suggest that isoflavones in soy reduce the risk of prostate, breast and colon cancer. The mechanisms for the action of the isoflavones are not clear, but they may work in the early stages of cancer development, perhaps by acting as anti-estrogens. More research is needed, both in the area of cancer prevention and also regarding the role soyfoods play in helping prevent the progression of these cancers.

The National Cancer Institute and the University of California, Los Angeles, are two institutions studying prostate cancer and the effects of diet, especially a diet rich in soyfoods.

Soy for Your Bones

Osteoporosis is a serious disorder in which bones become porous and brittle because of calcium loss. It is a major health problem today, particularly among older women in North America. Women in Asia, however, do not suffer osteoporosis in such high numbers. That fact has led scientists to suspect there may be a connection between diet and osteoporosis, particularly in the consumption of soy products.

Research supports this notion. Scientists are finding that eating soy may benefit our bones in two ways:

1. People who eat soy protein seem to *lose less calcium* through the urine than they would if they ate animal protein. This finding suggests that people who eat soy probably retain more calcium in their bodies.

2. People who consume isoflavones in soy products may *retain more calcium in the bones* themselves than they might otherwise.

In addition to the benefits soy protein and the isoflavones provide, many soyfoods are excellent sources of calcium (see section on Calcium and Soy, page xix).

From what scientists know today, soy can help prevent osteoporosis. For the greatest benefit, eat soyfoods high in both protein *and* isoflavones.

To Flash or Not to Flash

Isoflavones are considered "weak estrogens." They represent a possible alternative to hormone replacement therapy in postmenopausal women, particularly those who cannot or choose not to take estrogen supplements. Asian women seem to experience fewer hot flashes than Western women do. This may be the effect of a high soy diet, but more research is needed to determine if soy provides the real answer. In several studies under way at present, researchers are trying to determine if soy is truly helpful in controlling the symptoms of menopause, and if it is, to what degree.

Phytoestrogens

Because its chemical structure is similar to that of the hormone estrogen, isoflavones are often called *plant estrogens*. They act like weak estrogens in the body. They may increase bone density and reduce the intensity of hot flashes.

What about Soyfood Allergies?

A small percentage of people are allergic to soy protein. Soyfoods that have been fermented, such as miso or tempeh, and foods that have been heated during production reduce the incidence of such problems. However, anyone who is allergic to soy protein should read labels carefully to determine if it has been added to processed foods such as baked goods or beverages, either as a nutritional supplement or just as an ingredient to add moisture.

How Much Soy Should I Eat?

The latest recommendations for soyfoods range from one to three servings per day. The amount of soy protein and isoflavones you will need to consume depends on the benefits you are looking for and your general health. For those in good health, one serving of a food that provides 8 to 10 grams of soy protein and 16 to 20 milligrams of soy isoflavones per day (on average) is sufficient. Those with osteoporosis, diabetes or other risk factors for heart disease may want to eat more. Individuals with heart disease may want to eat four servings of soyfoods (25 milligrams) to help in efforts to reverse the disease. However, individuals making major changes to their diet should do so only with the knowledge and consent of their healthcare provider.

Soy portion sizes for children are similar to those of other foods, based on the child's age and activity level. Many infants are fed formulas based on soy milk. Unless there is a soy allergy, feeding children soyfoods is a good idea and may help prevent heart disease or cancer when they become adults.

For those in good health, one serving of a food that provides 8 to 10 grams of soy protein and 16 to 20 milligrams of soy isoflavones per day (on average) is sufficient.

Soy protein. An overview of soy's health benefits made by Dr. James Anderson at the University of Kentucky finds that significant reductions (10 to 15%) in total blood cholesterol, LDL and triglyceride levels occur with an average consumption of 47 grams of soy protein per day. A person who wishes to consume that much soy protein needs to eat at least four servings of soy products or two soy drinks each day.

One adult serving of soyfoods equals

1/2 cup tofu
1 cup soy milk
1/2 cup (2 ounces) crumbled tempeh
1/2 cup cooked soybeans

Soy Protein in Common Soyfoods

Soyfood	Soy Protein
8 oz. soy milk	7 grams
1/2 cup firm tofu	18 grams
1/2 cup cooked green soybeans	11 grams
1 oz. (1/3 cup) protein-isolate product (used in fruit drinks)	approximately 25 grams

On November 10, 1998, the Food and Drug Administration (FDA) announced it was considering allowing a health claim for the cholesterol-lowering properties of soy protein. In order to carry this claim on its label, a food product would have to contain at least 6.25 grams of soy protein per serving. This amount is based on the assumption that 25 grams of soy protein per day significantly lowers serum cholesterol levels and that an individual could eat four servings per day.

Foods that contain at least 6.25 grams per day would include 1 cup soy milk, 1/4 cup firm tofu, 1/3 cup cooked soybeans or 2 tablespoons soy protein isolates (soy powder).

Isoflavones. Soyfoods contain varying amounts of isoflavones. Many soyfood products now identify the isoflavone amounts per serving on their labels. Tofu, soy milk, soy flour, soynuts and textured soy protein are the best sources. One serving of these foods provides 30 to 40 milligrams of isoflavones.

Isolated soy protein and soy-protein concentrate vary in isoflavone content depending on the method used to extract them from soybeans. As a rule, levels in soy-protein concentrates (often the soy in soy burgers, for example) are very low. Soy sauce and soy oil contain *no* isoflavones at all.

Where to Purchase Soyfoods

Most supermarkets sell tofu and meat alternatives. Some carry soy milks, soy flour and textured soy protein. Look for soyfoods such as tofu and soy cream cheese in the produce section (remember, they are vegetables!). Sometimes the tofu and soy beverages are in the refrigerated sections. Others, such as the green soybeans and soynut butter, are found in the frozen-food cases. Some products, such as canned soybeans, soynut butter and shelf-stable soy beverages, are found on supermarket shelves. Natural-food stores sell soynuts, soynut butter and tempeh.

Some soyfoods are available by mail order. See page 153 for more information.

Soyfoods are in supermarkets everywhere, but if you don't see your favorite products, *ask for them*—and then make a point of expressing your appreciation when they appear. The supermarket won't know you want it unless you create the demand. Asking for what you want is the best way to ensure a steady supply.

How to Add Soy to Your Diet

Making the transition to a diet that is higher in soyfoods is easy! Here are tips that can help:

* Start slowly, just as you should when adding any new food to your menus. Soybeans *are* beans, so soy products can cause flatulence if you start eating them in large quantities suddenly. With time, your system will adapt and you will handle the higher amounts more readily. Supplements to help prevent gas formation are available if you need them. Ask your pharmacist.

* Add small amounts of TSP (textured soy protein) or tofu to your usual casseroles and stews. If you don't announce the change to your family, they probably won't notice the difference.

* Substitute soy protein—either as drained, crumbled tofu or textured soy protein (TSP)—for about one-quarter of the meat in meat dishes, such as meat loaf. Later you might want to increase the amount to one-third or one-half.

* Add a meat alternate, such as soy sausage, to familiar recipes that contain several ingredients. The change will be less obvious than if you served the product by itself.

* Substitute puréed tofu for sour cream in dips, sauces and dressings. (Puréeing also eliminates the white specks that announce tofu as one of the ingredients.)

* Add small amounts of soy flour to baked goods. Start with 1 tablespoon in every cup of all-purpose flour.

* Use soy milk in baking or in blended drinks.

* Try different soy milk brands to find your personal favorite. Flavor and texture vary dramatically from brand to brand.

❀ Use soynut butter on sandwiches. It has about the same amount of fat as reduced-fat peanut butter.

❀ Add silken tofu to blended fruit drinks.

❀ Substitute canned soybeans and frozen green soybeans for a portion of the beans called for in a bean salad, soup or casserole.

❀ Add frozen green soybeans directly to soups and side dishes. They cook in about 10 minutes.

Important Notes about Eating Soy

Soyfoods are part of a balanced diet. Remember, make soyfoods part of a *balanced diet* that includes a variety of fruits, vegetables and whole grains. You may consume soyfoods in addition to—or as a replacement for—some meats and dairy foods. Because soyfoods are high in protein and contain no cholesterol, you might want to include some meatless soy meals in your diet.

Most soyfoods do contain fat. Many soyfoods are high in fat, but most of it is polyunsaturated fat. (This is an important distinction because only saturated fatty acids and dietary cholesterol raise blood-cholesterol levels, which contributes to atherosclerosis and heart disease.) However, a soyfood high in fat content is a soyfood high in calories! If you are watching your weight, high calories are a concern for you. You can buy some products, such as soy milk, in fat-free and reduced-fat versions. Reduced-fat tofu is also available. Textured soy protein (TSP) is fat-free; use it as a substitute for some of the ground meat you would normally add to your favorite recipes.

Eat soyfoods, not supplements. Research concerning the different phytochemicals and nutrients in soybeans is in progress; we don't know everything about how soy exerts its effects on our health. Some soy components may work best in certain combinations, while other substances in soy may be beneficial all by themselves. Until we know more, play it safe and enjoy soy as a food—such as tofu, soy milk and TSP—and not in supplement form.

Get calcium from soy. Many soyfoods are a good source of calcium. A calcium compound is added during production, as in some types of tofu, or the product is fortified with calcium, as in some soy milks, or the food, such as whole soybeans, naturally contains calcium. One cup of cooked, mature soybeans has about 175 milligrams of calcium and one cup of cooked green soybeans has about 260 milligrams of calcium. (For comparison, one cup of cows' milk has about 300 milligrams.)

The body can absorb and use calcium from soy to about the same degree as it uses calcium from cows' milk. Unlike animal protein, soy protein may also help the body *retain* the calcium that is eaten by reducing urinary loss. In addition, the isoflavones in soy may prevent calcium loss from bone.

It's important to have calcium sources besides cows' milk, because about 80% of the world's population is *lactase insufficient*. People who are lactase insufficient can't completely digest milk sugar (lactose), because the enzyme necessary for that is not available in a sufficient amount. Vegetables and grains can contribute some calcium, but the amount from those sources is small compared to milk. Soy milk that has been fortified with calcium can be a significant source of this mineral, particularly for those who cannot consume cows' milk.

To determine how much calcium is in a soyfood, read the part of the package label under Nutrition Facts. Calcium content is listed as a percentage of the Dietary

Reference Intake (DRI) for calcium, which is 1000 milligrams (mg). For example, if the amount listed is "Calcium—10%," multiply 1000mg by 0.10 to determine the milligrams of calcium per serving (in this case, 100mg).

Do not take a calcium supplement with a meal high in soy. Substances called *phytates* in soy attach to calcium and prevent the body from absorbing it properly. Fermented soy products, such as miso and tempeh, have less of these substances than nonfermented soyfoods.

Soy and sodium. Consuming sodium in the diet affects the blood pressure of certain sodium-sensitive people. Some soy products, such as miso and soy sauces (even reduced-sodium soy sauce), are high in sodium. Use these products sparingly if you are on a low-sodium diet. Read labels on all soyfoods to determine if the sodium level is appropriate for you.

Cook before eating. Raw soybeans contain a substance that prevents dietary protein from being digested normally. Soybeans should be cooked before eating, because cooking soybeans destroys more than 90% of this substance, which is called a *protease inhibitor*. The remaining amount is not enough to affect protein digestion and actually may be important in preventing several kinds of cancer.

Don't Self-Treat

Don't make major changes to your diet in the hope of obtaining a certain health benefit without first consulting your physician, dietitian or other health professional who knows your medical history. That person should advise you, but also he or she should know how your diet has changed, because it may affect other areas of your care.

Do not *replace any of your prescription drugs with soyfoods until instructed to do so by your physician.*

A Soyfoods Glossary

The more processing the soyfood undergoes (the further from the plain bean) beyond what is necessary to make soy flour, tofu, canned soybeans and soy protein isolate, the less of the beneficial elements of soy may be contained in the food. Make sure the soyfoods you buy actually do contain a high percentage of soy.

It's an exciting time to be "going soy," because more products are available and soyfoods are better than ever before. Flavors have improved, and soyfoods are available in all kinds of products that are easier than ever to use in your favorite recipes. Major supermarkets now stock soyfoods routinely, and so do natural-food stores and Asian markets. You are sure to find items that will appeal to you and your family. Children will particularly like the soynut butter with jelly for a sandwich, or roasted soynuts—perhaps mixed with dried fruit—for a healthful snack.

The following information describes the wide variety of soyfoods you will find available. It also will help you learn to read labels efficiently, which will make buying soyfoods even easier. Check page 153 for mail-order sources.

Black Soybeans and Yellow Soybeans

These beans are both available either dried or canned. Canned soybeans offer an advantage because they require a much shorter cooking time. Black soybeans are lower in both protein and fat than the more common yellow soybeans.

Dried soybeans. Soak dried soybeans before cooking them. Dried soybeans require a longer cooking time than most other dried beans—see page 78. Cooking them in a pressure cooker speeds up the process. The longer the soybeans have been stored, the more cooking time they will require, so buy the beans from a store that has a rapid turnover in stock if possible. After soaking, you can roast them—see *Soynuts*, page xxvi.

Canned Soybeans. Drain and rinse the canned black soybeans before use. The liquid in canned yellow soybeans has a gel-like consistency. To remove it, just put the beans in a strainer and rinse off the liquid under running water. Then add the beans as usual to salads, casseroles and other dishes. They work well in almost any recipe that calls for cooked or canned dried beans. One producer, Eden Foods, cans black soybeans without salt.

Green Soybeans (Edamamé)

Use green soybeans in any recipe that calls for beans. Harvested at about 80% maturity, green soybeans are high in protein and fiber. Green soybeans are one of my favorite soyfoods. They are somewhat similar to green lima beans, but with a better flavor—to my taste—and a firmer texture. Usually sold in the pod, they are boiled for 15 to 20 minutes before shelling. Also called *sweet beans*, shelled green soybeans are available frozen.

> Green soybeans are high in protein and fiber.

Meat Alternatives or Analogs

Meat alternatives, or analogs, are soy products that resemble meat products in look and taste. To make a meat analog, soy protein, tofu and other ingredients are mixed with flavorings. Meat alternatives are sold as frozen, refrigerated or dried products. They are convenient to use; however, read labels to see how they fit into your diet because the ingredients vary.

Miso

Miso is a smooth, salty paste made from four ingredients: soybeans, a grain such as rice or barley, salt and a mold culture. Aged in wooden vats for one to two years, miso is used in small amounts as a seasoning agent or to make soups. Miso comes in several flavors. Usually the lighter the color, the milder the taste. Store miso in the refrigerator; it will keep for several months that way. When you add miso to a recipe, you do not need to add salt.

Soy Cheeses

Soy cheeses are available in flavors similar to regular cheeses, but in consistency they are more like a processed cheese than an aged, firm Cheddar. Soy cheeses containing *caseinate*, a milk protein, melt smoothly. Use them to make sauces and grilled-cheese sandwiches. Some soy cheeses seem to clump when mixed with an acid, such as canned tomatoes, so you may need to experiment a little to see what works best in your own recipes.

Soy cream cheese is also available. It works well in dips and desserts. It has a beany taste that disappears when it is mixed with other ingredients and the flavors are given time to blend. Soy cream cheese is pale tan in color.

Soy Flour

Ground from roasted soybeans, soy flour is a fine powder. You can buy it in two forms: natural (full-fat) and defatted. In baked goods, you may replace up to one-fourth of the wheat flour called for with soy flour. Always stir soy flour before measuring.

Because soy flour contains no gluten—the protein in wheat that enables baked goods to rise—products made with soy flour have a denser texture. When adding soy flour, start by adding 1 to 2 tablespoons. Each time you make the recipe, substitute a little more soy flour for the wheat flour (up to no more than one-fifth), until you find the proportion that gives you the finished baked good you want.

Store soy flour in the refrigerator.

Tip: To reduce cholesterol in baking, replace one egg with 1 tablespoon soy flour and 1 tablespoon water.

Soy Grits

Soy grits are similar to soy flour but have a coarser texture. Soy grits are used in baking, casseroles and grain dishes. When added to casseroles, they absorb moisture during cooking and have a texture that is somewhat similar to cooked bulghur.

Soy Milk (Soy Beverages)

Even though it is widely known as *soy milk*, this product will be found in the market as *soy beverage* because of federal labeling guidelines. Soy milk is available plain and flavored. Read labels carefully! "Plain" in this case does *not* usually mean "unsweetened." Almost all soy milks contain some type of sweetener, often barley or brown-rice syrup. Use these sweetened milks for drinking, on breakfast cereals and for desserts and quick breads. Soy milks are available in reduced-fat, fat-free and full-fat versions.

If you can't find soy milk in the refrigerated section of your grocery store, look for it near the canned milks. Soy milk is usually packaged in shelf-stable containers. After opening the container, store soy milk in the refrigerator for up to 5 days.

Soybean Oil

Mostly composed of polyunsaturated fatty acids, soybean oil is the most widely used cooking oil in the United States. It does not confer the health benefits of soy protein or isoflavones. However, it does contain large amounts of polyunsaturated fat.

Soynuts

A good source of protein, fiber and isoflavones, soynuts are available in several flavors.

Similar to peanuts, soynuts are whole dried soybeans that have been soaked in water and are either fried or roasted in oil until browned and crunchy. A good source of protein, fiber and isoflavones, soynuts are available in several flavors. You can make your own—see page 82. They are sometimes called *roasted soybeans*.

Soynut Butter (Roasted Soybean Butter)

Ground or crushed roasted soynuts are mixed with soybean oil and other ingredients to make a spread that can be used for sandwiches or in cooking. Soynut butter is similar to soynuts in its nutritional content, but soynut butter is higher in fat. More than half the calories in soynut butter are fat calories.

Soy Protein Concentrates
Soy protein concentrate contains about 70% protein but also has the soybean's dietary fiber. It is made from defatted soy flakes. Soy protein concentrate is used in manufactured foods such as vegetable burgers and baked goods; check the label. It is not as rich in isoflavones as soy protein isolates.

Soy Protein Isolates
The most highly refined form of soy protein, isolates are 92% protein. They are made from defatted soy flakes. Isolates are used in a wide range of commercially prepared foods, including infant and nutritional formulas, breads, cereals and baked goods. They are available as a powder for use as a food supplement. The powder is sold in natural-food stores as *soy protein* or *soy powder*; check the label to ensure that you are buying soy protein isolates and not the concentrate.

Soy Sauces (Tamari, Shoyu)
Tamari, a by-product of miso production, is made only from soybeans, while shoyu contains wheat and soybeans. Both are the result of fermentation. Salty in flavor, soy sauces contain none of the health benefits of other soy products. Reduced-sodium soy sauce is available.

Soy Yogurt

Soy yogurt is made from soy milk. Use it in place of sour cream or regular yogurt. Like regular yogurt, it is available plain or flavored. Soy yogurt is darker in color than yogurt made from cows' milk, so it may affect the color of some dishes.

Tempeh

Probably one of the least known soyfoods to Westerners, tempeh is a traditional Indonesian product. Soybeans, with or without grains, are combined with a food-grade mold that binds the beans and grains together into a cake. Some people say the flavor of tempeh reminds them of mushrooms.

Tempeh is a good source of vitamin B12. It is available in natural-food stores either refrigerated or frozen. Tempeh is usually steamed for about 20 minutes before being crumbled or cut into pieces for use in sandwiches, salads or main dishes. Sometimes I use it as the main ingredient, and I also add it to a small amount of cooked chicken when making salads or sandwiches. It goes particularly well with curry flavors.

Tempeh can be frozen for several months or refrigerated for about a week.

Tempeh is a good source of vitamin B12.

Textured Soy Protein (TSP)

TSP is made from soy flour that has been changed by cooking and extruding it. This is the pale, dry, chunky or granular product that we find in natural-food stores called a *meat extender* or *meat substitute*. When mixed with boiling water, TSP resembles the texture of ground meat but is lighter in color. If you use seasonings that add color, it looks even more like meat. It contains about 70% protein and is a good source of fiber. TVP® (Textured Vegetable Protein), which is widely available,

TSP is a good source of fiber.

is the registered-trademark brand of the Archer Daniels Midland Company.

TSP can be stored at room temperature for several months. Once TSP is rehydrated, refrigerate it and use it within 2 or 3 days.

Tofu

Whole books have been written about tofu! Here is a quick review of this versatile food.

Tofu is made from soy milk, much as cheese is made from milk. Two common agents are used to coagulate soy milk into tofu. They are *nigari* (magnesium chloride) or calcium sulfate. Some feel that tofu made from nigari is superior, but the kind made with calcium is a good source of that mineral, which is deficient in many diets. The coagulating agent used is listed in the ingredients list on the label. Read more about calcium and soy on page xix.

Tofu is probably the most versatile of the soyfoods and one of the easiest ways to increase the amount of soy you eat. It contains the important soy protein and isoflavones. All it lacks is fiber. Protein and fat content vary according to the firmness of the tofu. Protein content is usually highest in the firmer tofu. Fat content usually *decreases* as softness *increases*.

Regular and silken tofu. Tofu comes in two basic types—regular and silken. *Regular tofu* is usually packaged with water in 16- or 19-ounce containers and must be refrigerated. It is available as *soft, firm* and *extra-firm*. Use regular tofu in stir-fries, soups and sandwiches. After opening, replace the water, cover and use within a week, changing the water daily.

Silken tofu, also available as *soft, firm* and *extra-firm*, has a creamy texture. It is used in dips, sauces and

> Tofu is made from soy milk, much as cheese is made from milk.

desserts. Silken tofu, both full-fat and reduced-fat, is often available in 12-ounce packages with an extended shelf life. Refrigerate after opening and use within 3 days.

Preparation: Seasoning, draining and even disguising tofu. Tofu can be crumbled, mashed, sliced, diced and even frozen. Blended with chocolate, tofu becomes a dessert. Add garlic, lemon juice and herbs, and it is a tasty dip for raw vegetables or chips. Because tofu has a bland flavor and a porous texture, it absorbs seasonings readily. You may have to over-season tofu somewhat to get the flavor you want.

After you open the package, always drain tofu well. Press tofu that has been packaged in water between paper towels to remove more of the liquid. Draining and pressing the tofu will help ensure your dips or sauces have the proper consistency. Otherwise they may be too thin.

To prevent small white specks from appearing in sauces and baked goods, I prefer to purée the tofu in a food processor before adding it to a recipe. The white specks give away your secret that tofu was used in the recipe *and* that the dish may actually be good for your family or guests.

Tofu is available smoked, baked and fried. You may use these tasty versions for salads and sandwiches without additional seasoning.

Freezing tofu. Water-packed tofu can remain frozen for up to 5 months. Defrost in the package in the refrigerator or in a pan of cold water. Drain and press out the moisture. The tofu's texture will resemble a sponge. Shred the tofu before use. Defrosted tofu is drier than "regular" tofu. It is a good choice when you must be careful not to add too much moisture to a recipe, such as "meat" balls, burgers or spreads.

Spongy, defrosted tofu absorbs marinades or dressings quickly and efficiently.

appetizers

RECIPES IN THIS CHAPTER RANGE FROM easy-to-make dips to an elegant filo pastry that would be a perfect first course at any party. Because appetizers are served in small portions, they are a good way to introduce soy products to your family and friends. In most of the dishes, the soy ingredient is in disguise. Guests won't know they're eating nutritious soy.

TIP

Need an easy dip? Add 2 cups puréed, well-drained, reduced-fat firm tofu to a package of ranch dressing or onion soup mix and stir to combine. Let the dip stand for a few minutes before serving so the flavors can develop.

Roasted Bell Pepper & Tofu Spread

If you don't want to roast your own, buy roasted bell peppers packed in jars. Drain them well before using. Leftover bell peppers are delicious on sandwiches or in salads.

2 red bell peppers, roasted, peeled, seeds and core removed and chopped

2 large garlic cloves, minced

1 cup (8 oz.) extra-firm silken tofu, drained

½ cup (4 oz.) goat cheese

1 tablespoon fresh lemon juice or to taste

1 tablespoon balsamic vinegar

½ teaspoon salt

½ teaspoon coarsely ground black pepper

Hot pepper sauce to taste

Crackers, crudités or bread sticks, to serve

Place the bell peppers, garlic, tofu and goat cheese in a food processor or blender. Process until smooth. Season with lemon juice, vinegar, salt, pepper and hot pepper sauce. Cover and refrigerate 30 minutes for flavors to blend.

Serve with crackers, crudités or bread sticks.

❋ Makes about 1-3/4 cups.

❋ 2 tablespoons contain:

Cal 57	Prot 4g	Carb 2g
Fat 3.8g	Chol 6mg	Sodium 120mg

Note:
Roasting Bell Peppers and Chiles

Pierce each bell pepper or green chile with the tip of a knife. Grill or broil until blistered and blackened on all sides. Place peppers in a bowl that holds them snugly and cover bowl with plastic wrap. The steam that collects helps loosen the skins. Let stand until cool enough to handle. Peel peppers and remove cores and seeds. Cut into strips, chop or leave whole for stuffing.

If you have an abundance of red bell peppers or green chiles, you may freeze them after grilling, but don't peel them. They are even easier to peel after freezing.

Southwestern Hummus
see page 12

Chicken-Green Chile Stew
see page 17

Blue Cheese & Tofu Spread

If you like a pungent blue cheese with lots of flavor, use Roquefort cheese from the caves of southwestern France or Stilton cheese from England.

Combine all ingredients except crackers in a food processor or blender. Process until smooth. Cover and refrigerate 30 minutes to enable flavors to blend.

Serve with crackers, crudités or pita bread cut into triangular pieces for dipping.

❋ Makes 3/4 cup.

❋ 2 tablespoons contain:
Cal 63	Prot 5g	Carb 2g
Fat 4g	Chol 7mg	Sodium 134mg

2 garlic cloves, minced

½ cup (4 oz.) extra-firm silken tofu, drained

¼ cup blue cheese, softened

½ teaspoon freshly ground black pepper

1 tablespoon fresh lemon juice or to taste

Crackers, crudités or pita bread, to serve

Artichoke-Stuffed Mushrooms

Enjoy these hot, tender morsels as an appetizer or first course.

8 to 10 large
   mushrooms

2 teaspoons olive oil

2 tablespoons
   minced onion

2 tablespoons
   finely chopped
   red bell pepper

¾ cup (6 oz.) firm
   tofu, drained

1 (15-oz.) can
   quartered
   artichoke hearts,
   drained and rinsed

¼ to ½ cup dried
   breadcrumbs

½ teaspoon dried
   oregano

2 tablespoons fresh
   lemon juice

½ teaspoon salt

Freshly ground
   black pepper

4 tablespoons
   freshly grated
   Parmesan cheese

Preheat oven to 375F (190C). Spray a large baking pan with nonstick cooking spray. Wipe mushrooms with a damp paper towel and remove stems. Chop stems.

Heat oil in a nonstick skillet over medium heat. Add onion, chopped stems and bell pepper. Cook, stirring occasionally, until browned and liquid evaporates.

Meanwhile, process tofu in a food processor until smooth. Add artichoke hearts and mushroom mixture and process until coarsely chopped.

Stir in breadcrumbs, oregano, lemon juice, salt and pepper. Arrange mushroom caps in prepared pan. Spoon artichoke mixture into mushroom caps, mounding slightly. Sprinkle with Parmesan cheese. Bake about 10 minutes or until mushrooms are tender and topping is browned.

❋ Makes 4 servings.

❋ 1 serving contains:
   Cal 195   Prot 14g   Carb 18g
   Fat 8g   Chol 5mg   Sodium 755mg

Dilled Salmon Spread

Make this ahead to allow time for the superb flavors to blend. If dill is not your favorite seasoning, use an equal amount of tarragon or chives instead.

Combine all ingredients except salmon in a food processor and process until smooth. Add salmon and pulse until combined but still chunky. Cover and refrigerate 30 minutes for flavors to blend. Serve with French Bread Crisps and crudités.

❀ Makes about 2 cups.

❀ 2 tablespoons contain:

Cal 36	Prot 4g	Carb 1g
Fat 2g	Chol 9mg	Sodium 93mg

French Bread Crisps

Cut a loaf of French bread into ¼-inch-thick slices. Arrange slices in one layer on a large baking sheet. Bake in a preheated 350F (175C) oven for 10 to 15 minutes or until lightly toasted. Cool and store in an airtight container.

¾ cup (6 oz.) extra-firm low-fat silken tofu, drained

4 oz. whipped low-fat cream cheese

2 tablespoons chopped fresh dill or 1 tablespoon dried

2 teaspoons prepared horseradish

1 teaspoon Dijon mustard

1 (6-oz.) can boneless, skinless salmon, drained

French Bread Crisps (see opposite) and crudités, to serve

Easy Tuna Dip

When unexpected guests arrive, you can make this recipe quickly from ingredients in your pantry and refrigerator. Serve as a dip, pita filling or sandwich spread.

½ cup (4 oz.) extra-firm silken tofu, drained

1 (15-oz.) can quartered artichoke hearts, drained and rinsed

1 (6-oz.) can water-packed tuna, drained

1 tablespoon minced fresh tarragon, or 1 teaspoon dried

2 tablespoons fresh lemon juice

Dash of hot pepper sauce or to taste

Process tofu in a food processor until smooth. Add artichoke hearts and process until coarsely chopped. Add tuna, tarragon, lemon juice and hot pepper sauce and pulse just to combine; mixture should be chunky. Cover and refrigerate 30 minutes for flavors to blend.

❋ Makes about 2-½ cups.

❋ 2 tablespoons contain:
Cal 22   Prot 3g   Carb 2g
Fat 0g   Chol 2mg   Sodium 48mg

Tip: Unopened 12-ounce packages of silken tofu have a long shelf life. However, when using less than the full package, refrigerate the unused portions in an air-tight container and use within two days.

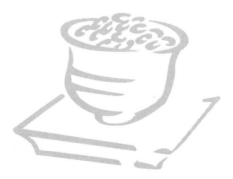

Roasted Eggplant Spread

Roasting vegetables adds a new depth of flavor to dishes containing them. Almost any vegetable can be roasted for more flavor; the root vegetables are particularly good.

Preheat oven to 350F (175C). Spray a nonstick roasting pan with nonstick cooking spray. Arrange eggplant, onion, tomatoes and garlic in prepared pan. Roast tomatoes and garlic about 30 minutes or until soft and remove. Roast eggplant and onion about 15 minutes longer or until soft. Cool vegetables, peel and coarsely chop and place in a medium bowl.

Meanwhile, steam tempeh in a steamer basket over boiling water 20 minutes. Remove from steamer and cool. Add tempeh to vegetables.

Stir vinegar, sesame oil, capers, salt and pepper into vegetable mixture and stir to combine. Cover and refrigerate 30 minutes for flavors to blend. Serve with pita bread.

❈ Makes about 4 cups.

❈ 2 tablespoons contain:
Cal 25	Prot 2g	Carb 3g
Fat 1g	Chol 0mg	Sodium 54mg

1 (about 1-lb.) eggplant

1 small onion, cut in half crosswise

4 plum tomatoes, cut in half lengthwise

4 garlic cloves (unpeeled)

1 (8-oz.) package soy tempeh, crumbled

2 tablespoons balsamic vinegar

1 tablespoon sesame oil

1 tablespoon capers, minced

½ teaspoon salt

Coarsely ground black pepper

Pita bread, to serve

Smoked Salmon Rolls

Serve these pretty pink-and-white spirals at your next party.

¼ cup (2 oz.) extra-firm low-fat silken tofu, drained

1 (8-oz.) package soy cream cheese

1 tablespoon chopped fresh tarragon, or 2 teaspoons dried

1 tablespoon prepared horseradish

2 tablespoons fresh lemon juice

About 4 oz. smoked salmon slices

Tarragon sprigs, to garnish

Process tofu and cream cheese in a food processor until smooth. Stir in tarragon, horseradish and lemon juice. Cover and refrigerate 30 minutes.

Separate salmon into individual slices on a cutting board. Divide filling mixture among salmon slices. Roll salmon slices, starting at a short side, to enclose filling. Place on a plate, cover and refrigerate until chilled.

To serve, cut rolls crosswise with a serrated knife into 2-inch pieces. Garnish with tarragon sprigs.

❈ Makes 6 servings.

❈ 1 serving contains:
Cal 139   Prot 6g   Carb 3g
Fat 12g   Chol 4mg   Sodium 424mg

Variation
Substitute dill for the tarragon.

Crab Quesadillas with Avocado Sauce

For a taste of Mexico, try these! Golden and crisp on the outside, they are creamy and delicious on the inside. Choose soy cheese that lists caseinate (a dairy product) as one of the ingredients to ensure it will melt easily.

Prepare Avocado Sauce (see below) and refrigerate.

Heat a griddle over medium heat. Place 2 tortillas on hot griddle. Divide crabmeat and cheese between tortillas. Sprinkle with cilantro, if using. Top with remaining tortillas.

Cook, turning once, until tortillas are browned and cheese is melted, about 3 minutes. Cut quesadillas into wedges. Serve with Avocado Sauce.

❈ Makes 16 wedges.

❈ 1 wedge with sauce contains:

Cal 70	Prot 4g	Carb 5g
Fat 4g	Chol 6mg	Sodium 126mg

Avocado Sauce

Peel avocado and cut into pieces. Process avocado and tofu in a food processor until smooth. Add lemon juice and process to combine. Stir in chile. Cover and refrigerate until served.

❈ Makes 1-½ cups.

Note: Remove the seeds from the chile if you want to reduce the heat. It's a good idea to wear rubber gloves when chopping hot chiles to prevent the oil from irritating your hands.

QUESADILLAS:

4 (about 7-inch) flour tortillas

4 oz. flaked crabmeat

4 oz. Monterey jack-style soy cheese, finely chopped

2 tablespoons chopped cilantro leaves (optional)

AVOCADO SAUCE:

1 small ripe avocado

½ cup (4 oz.) silken tofu, drained

2 tablespoons fresh lemon juice

1 jalapeño chile, minced

Vegetable-Cheese Filo Slices

Tofu and feta cheese are blended with the vegetables to add protein and flavor to this special appetizer. For variety, try using feta with herbs and sun-dried tomatoes.

1 tablespoon soft margarine

1 cup finely chopped onion

2 cups finely chopped green cabbage

1 large garlic clove, minced

1 teaspoon dried marjoram

1 teaspoon cumin seeds

1 cup (8 oz.) extra-firm low-fat tofu, drained

4 oz. feta cheese, crumbled

10 to 12 filo pastry sheets

About ¼ cup soft margarine, melted

Preheat oven to 375F (190C). Spray a baking sheet with nonstick cooking spray. Melt margarine in a large skillet over medium heat. Add onion, cover and cook, stirring occasionally, 5 minutes. Add cabbage and garlic, cover and cook, stirring occasionally, until crisp-tender, about 5 minutes. Stir in marjoram and cumin seeds. Cool slightly.

Process tofu in a food processor until smooth. Stir in feta cheese. Stir tofu mixture into vegetable mixture in skillet.

Place 1 filo sheet on a work surface and cover remaining pastry with plastic wrap to prevent drying. Brush filo sheet very lightly with melted margarine and top with another sheet of pastry. Continue with remaining pastry sheets and margarine.

Spoon filling along a long side of pastry. Fold in ends and roll to enclose filling. Place roll on prepared baking sheet and brush top with margarine. Bake about 30 minutes or until golden brown.

To serve, cut crosswise with a serrated knife into 1-½-inch pieces. Serve warm.

❀ Makes about 10 servings.

❀ 1 serving contains:
Cal 176   Prot 6g   Carb 16g
Fat 10g   Chol 10mg   Sodium 306mg

Variation

To save fat calories, spray the filo sheets with cooking spray instead of brushing with margarine. The pastry will still become golden, but will not be as crisp and will lose its crispness more quickly.

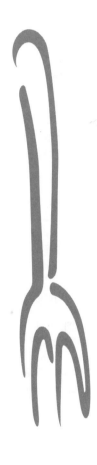

Southwestern Hummus

Hummus is a Middle-Eastern dish usually made with chickpeas and tahini. Here, two kinds of soybeans and Southwestern flavors are added. Stir in a touch of vegetable broth for a thinner dip.

1 (15-oz.) can yellow soybeans, drained and rinsed

1 (15-oz.) can black soybeans, drained and rinsed

¼ cup fresh parsley

2 large garlic cloves, minced

½ cup fresh lemon juice

1 tablespoon grated lemon zest

1 tablespoon mild ground red chile, or to taste

1 large tomato, chopped

1 serrano chile, minced

Baked tortilla chips, to serve

Process all ingredients, except tortilla chips, in the food processor until a good consistency for dipping. Transfer to a serving bowl. Serve with tortilla chips.

❈ Makes about 3 cups.

❈ 2 tablespoons contain:

Cal 41	Prot 5g	Carb 5g
Fat 2g	Chol 0mg	Sodium 22mg

Barbecued Tofu Bites

A piquant sauce is the perfect foil for tofu. Freezing makes the tofu more porous so it will easily absorb the sauce.

Drain tofu and squeeze to remove all moisture. Cut tofu lengthwise into 3 slices; set aside in a single layer in a shallow dish.

Combine tomato sauce, honey, vinegar, miso, sesame seeds, mustard and hot pepper sauce in a small bowl. Pour mixture over tofu, turn to coat both sides and let stand 15 minutes.

Preheat broiler. Spray a broiler pan with nonstick cooking spray. Arrange tofu on pan. Broil about 4 inches from heat until browned; turn and brown remaining side. Cut into cubes and serve with wooden picks.

❈ Makes 6 to 8 servings.

❈ 1 serving contains:

Cal 70	Prot 5g	Carb 10g
Fat 1.8g	Chol 0mg	Sodium 283mg

1 (16-oz.) package extra-firm tofu, frozen and thawed (page xxx)

½ cup tomato sauce

2 tablespoons honey

2 tablespoons cider vinegar

1 tablespoon white miso

1 tablespoon sesame seeds

1 teaspoon dry mustard

Hot pepper sauce to taste

soups

MAKING SOUPS IS AN EASY WAY TO USE SOY products. Tofu and soy milk, for example, can be used to make creamy soups without using cream. Miso paste adds rich flavor and can be used instead of salt. Miso is a nutritious product, with many B vitamins.

Add whole cooked soybeans to soups, stews and chilies. They add interest, texture and color as well as subtle flavor. Chicken–Green Chile Stew is a perfect example. Try it once and it will become a favorite. Using canned soybeans also saves cooking time.

You may use TSP (textured soy protein) instead of meat. You don't have to mix it with water before using if the TSP will be simmered in liquid along with other ingredients. Soy protein products that are already seasoned and formed into meat alternatives (to look like ground beef, for example) can also be used in soups.

Curried Pumpkin Soup

This is my favorite way to serve vitamin-rich pumpkin. It's better at Thanksgiving than pumpkin pie! This soup always receives raves, even from people who say they don't like soup or tofu.

1 tablespoon soft margarine or butter

½ cup chopped onion

½ cup chopped celery

1 garlic clove, minced

2 (14.5-oz.) cans vegetable or fat-free, reduced-sodium chicken broth

½ teaspoon salt or to taste

Freshly ground white pepper

1 cup (8 oz.) soft silken tofu

1 cup cooked or canned puréed pumpkin

About 1 cup plain, unsweetened soy milk

2 teaspoons curry powder

Melt margarine in a large saucepan over medium heat. Add onion, celery and garlic and cook, stirring occasionally, until vegetables are soft, about 5 minutes.

Add broth, salt and pepper, cover and simmer, stirring occasionally, until vegetables are tender, about 20 minutes. With a slotted spoon, transfer vegetables to a food processor, leaving broth in pan.

Add tofu to food processor and pulse until vegetables are finely chopped and tofu is smooth. Add pumpkin and process until combined.

Add pumpkin mixture, soy milk and curry powder to broth in saucepan and heat until hot, adding more soy milk if soup is too thick.

❋ Makes 4 servings.

❋ 1 serving contains:
| Cal 124 | Prot 10g | Carb 11g |
| Fat 5g | Chol 0mg | Sodium 659mg |

Chicken–Green Chile Stew

Canned black soybeans are a relatively new product. They are an easy way to add soy protein to your recipes.

Heat half of the olive oil in a large nonstick pan over medium heat. Add onion and cook, stirring occasionally, until softened, about 5 minutes. Remove onion with a slotted spoon. Add remaining oil, garlic and chicken and cook, stirring occasionally, until browned, about 5 minutes. Return onion to pan.

Add green chiles, tomatoes, broth, soybeans, ground chile, oregano, bay leaf and salt. Reduce heat, cover and simmer 20 minutes or until onion and chicken are tender. Discard bay leaf. Spoon into bowl and sprinkle with cilantro, if using.

❈ Makes 3 or 4 servings.

❈ 1 serving contains:
Cal 348   Prot 35g   Carb 32g
Fat 10g   Chol 45mg   Sodium 773mg

3 teaspoons olive oil

1 small onion, chopped

1 large garlic clove, minced

8 oz. boneless, skinless chicken breasts, finely chopped

4 mild green chiles, roasted, peeled and cut into strips (see page 2) or 1 (4-oz.) can whole green chiles, cut into strips

2 cups chopped tomatoes

1 (14.5-oz) can fat-free chicken broth

1 (15-oz.) can black soybeans, drained and rinsed

1-½ teaspoons ground mild chile

1 teaspoon dried oregano

1 bay leaf

½ teaspoon salt or to taste

Chopped cilantro leaves (optional)

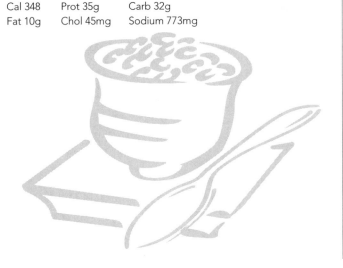

Shrimp Miso Soup

You'll be amazed at how quickly this delicate soup can be prepared. Don't boil the soup after you add the miso; just heat until hot.

1 teaspoon
  vegetable oil

2 green onions,
  including tops,
  finely chopped

1 garlic clove,
  minced

½ cup sliced
  mushrooms

1 teaspoon minced
  serrano chile
  (optional)

1 tablespoon
  red miso

2 cups vegetable
  broth or water

¼ cup small
  cooked peeled
  shrimp

Heat oil in a saucepan over medium heat. Add green onions, garlic, mushrooms and chile, if using. Cook, stirring, until vegetables are softened, 5 to 8 minutes.

In a small bowl, dissolve miso in ¼ of the broth. Add miso mixture, remaining broth and shrimp to saucepan. Do not boil; heat until hot, stirring occasionally.

❀ Makes 2 or 3 servings.

❀ 1 serving contains:
   Cal 80   Prot 8g   Carb 5g
   Fat 3g   Chol 55mg   Sodium 383mg

Variation
Substitute ½ cup cubed firm tofu for shrimp.

Leek & Potato Soup

Instead of being puréed in a food processor or blender, the vegetables are mashed with a potato masher or wooden spoon. Like the lumps in "real" mashed potatoes, this gives a comforting texture to the soup.

Cut root ends and darker green tops from leeks. Cut a lengthwise slit partially through each leek and rinse under running water to remove all sand. Thinly slice white and light-green parts of leeks.

Melt margarine in a large saucepan over low heat. Add leeks, onion and garlic, cover and cook, stirring occasionally, until leeks and onion are very soft, about 10 minutes.

Add potatoes, broth, bay leaf, thyme, salt and white pepper. Reduce heat, cover and simmer until potatoes are very tender, 15 to 20 minutes. Discard bay leaf and thyme sprig. Mash potatoes slightly with a potato masher or wooden spoon. Stir in soy milk and heat until hot. Garnish with chives, if desired.

❀ Makes 4 to 6 servings.

❀ 1 serving contains:
Cal 228   Prot 10g   Carb 40g
Fat 4g   Chol 0mg   Sodium 622mg

Variation

Omit salt and stir in 1 tablespoon white miso dissolved in 2 tablespoons hot water with soy milk.

2 large leeks

1 tablespoon soft margarine

1 cup thinly sliced onion

1 large garlic clove, minced

1 lb. russet potatoes, peeled and cut into small cubes

2 (14.5-oz.) cans fat-free, reduced-sodium chicken broth, or water

1 bay leaf

1 thyme sprig, or ¼ teaspoon dried

½ teaspoon salt or to taste

Freshly ground white pepper

1 cup plain, unsweetened soy milk

Minced chives (optional)

Salmon Chowder

You may add either cooked or canned salmon to this chowder. It has a particularly pleasing smoky flavor when made with leftover (or "planned-over"!) charcoal-grilled salmon.

1 tablespoon soft margarine or butter

½ cup finely chopped onion

1 medium leek, white and light-green parts only, finely chopped

½ cup finely chopped carrot

½ cup finely chopped celery

2 tablespoons finely chopped red bell pepper

1 lb. red potatoes, unpeeled, cut into small cubes

3 cups water or fat-free chicken broth

1 bay leaf

½ teaspoon salt or to taste

Freshly ground white pepper

6 oz. cooked or drained canned salmon, flaked

1 tablespoon minced fresh tarragon or 1 teaspoon dried

2 cups plain, unsweetened soy milk

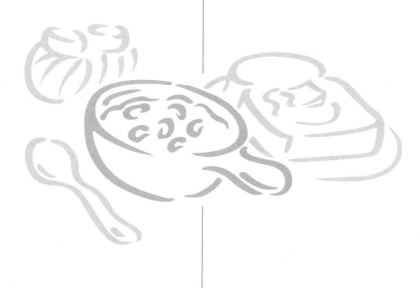

Melt margarine in a large saucepan over medium heat. Add onion, leek, carrot, celery and bell pepper and cook, stirring occasionally, until vegetables are soft, about 5 minutes.

Add potatoes, water, bay leaf, salt and white pepper. Reduce heat, cover and simmer until potatoes are tender, about 15 minutes. Discard bay leaf. Stir in salmon, tarragon and soy milk and heat until hot.

❀ Makes 4 servings.

❀ 1 serving contains:

Cal 177	Prot 18g	Carb 25g
Fat 8g	Chol 0mg	Sodium 332mg

Vegetable Soup

Adding soybeans to vegetable soups adds protein, so you can serve this as a main dish or as a first course. I like to top this soup with freshly grated Parmesan cheese.

2 teaspoons olive oil

1 cup chopped onion

1 cup chopped carrots

1 cup chopped celery

1 large garlic clove, minced

4 cups vegetable broth or water

1-¼ cups chopped red potatoes

2 cups chopped tomatoes

1 bay leaf

1 teaspoon dried basil

1 teaspoon dried thyme

½ teaspoon dried oregano

½ teaspoon salt or to taste

Freshly ground pepper

Dash of hot pepper sauce

1 cup chopped zucchini

1 cup shredded cabbage

1 cup sliced mushrooms

1 (15-oz.) can yellow soybeans, drained and rinsed

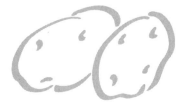

Heat oil in a large nonstick saucepan over low heat. Add onion, carrots, celery and garlic and cook, stirring occasionally, 5 minutes.

Add broth, potatoes, tomatoes, herbs, salt, pepper and hot pepper sauce. Cover and simmer until potatoes are almost tender, about 15 minutes. Discard bay leaf.

Add zucchini, cabbage, mushrooms and soybeans and simmer until vegetables are crisp-tender, about 10 minutes. Serve hot.

❈ Makes 6 servings.

❈ 1 serving contains:
| Cal 152 | Prot 13g | Carb 22g |
| Fat 2g | Chol 0mg | Sodium 539mg |

Creamy Broccoli Soup

Broccoli is so good for us that it should be the national vegetable! The tofu and potatoes make this delicious soup creamy without a touch of cream.

8 oz. russet potatoes, peeled and cut into small cubes

½ cup chopped onion

½ cup chopped celery

1 garlic clove, minced

2 (14.5-oz.) cans vegetable or fat-free chicken broth

1 (10-oz.) package frozen chopped broccoli

1 cup (8 oz.) soft silken tofu

About 1 cup plain, unsweetened soy milk

1 tablespoon white miso dissolved in 2 tablespoons

hot water

Bring potatoes, onion, celery, garlic and broth to a boil in a large saucepan. Reduce heat to low, cover and cook, stirring occasionally, 10 minutes.

Add broccoli and simmer, stirring occasionally, until vegetables are tender, about 10 minutes. With a slotted spoon transfer vegetables to a food processor, leaving broth in pan.

Add tofu to food processor and pulse until vegetables are finely chopped and tofu is smooth.

Add broccoli mixture, soy milk and miso mixture to broth in saucepan and heat until hot, adding more soy milk if soup is too thick.

❀ Makes 4 to 6 servings.

❀ 1 serving contains:
Cal 152   Prot 13g   Carb 22g
Fat 2g   Chol 0mg   Sodium 539mg

Black Soybean Soup

The pleasing flavor of miso adds an Asian touch to this Caribbean-style soup.

Combine all ingredients except miso and sherry in a large saucepan. Bring to a boil over medium heat. Reduce heat to low, cover and cook, stirring occasionally, until vegetables are tender, about 20 minutes.

Process soup in batches in a food processor until smooth. Return soup to saucepan and stir in miso mixture and sherry, if using. Heat until hot.

❊ Makes 4 to 6 cups.

❊ 1 serving contains:
Cal 272   Prot 24g   Carb 35g
Fat 3g   Chol 0mg   Sodium 478mg

2 (15-oz.) cans black soybeans, drained and rinsed

8 oz. russet potatoes, peeled and cut into small cubes

½ cup chopped onion

½ cup chopped celery

1 garlic clove, minced

2 (14.5-oz.) cans vegetable or fat-free chicken broth

Dash of hot pepper sauce

1 tablespoon red miso dissolved in 2 tablespoons hot water

2 tablespoons dry sherry (optional)

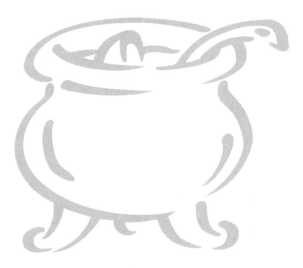

Crab Bisque

The anise-like flavor of tarragon complements seafood and chicken. It has a pronounced taste, so use it sparingly at first.

1 medium russet potato, peeled and diced

1 large leek, white and light-green parts only, finely chopped

½ cup chopped onion

½ cup chopped celery

1 small garlic clove, minced

½ teaspoon salt or to taste

4 cups water

½ cup (4 oz.) soft silken tofu

8 oz. flaked crabmeat

2 cups unsweetened plain soy milk

2 teaspoons minced fresh tarragon or ½ teaspoon dried

Dash of hot pepper sauce or to taste

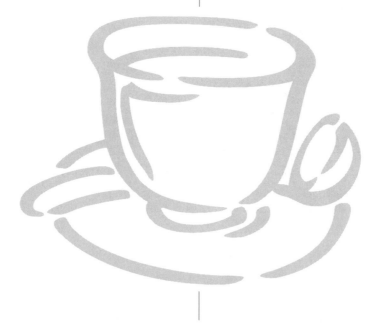

Bring potato, leek, onion, celery, garlic, salt and water to a boil in a large saucepan. Reduce heat to low, cover and cook, stirring occasionally, 20 minutes or until vegetables are tender.

With a slotted spoon, transfer vegetables to a food processor, leaving liquid in pan.

Add tofu to food processor and pulse until vegetables are finely chopped and tofu is smooth.

Add vegetable mixture, crabmeat, soy milk, tarragon and hot sauce to liquid in saucepan. Heat soup until hot, adding more soy milk if soup is too thick.

❋ Makes 6 servings.

❋ 1 serving contains:

Cal 125	Prot 12g	Carb 14g
Fat 2g	Chol 33mg	Sodium 340mg

Variation

Almost any cooked seafood can be substituted for the crab. This dish is also good made with shrimp or minced clams.

Black Bean Chili

Accompany this robust main dish with a mixed green salad and crusty cornbread. Because the seasonings are stirred directly into the turkey-TSP mix, they are absorbed more easily.

⅞ cup TSP (textured soy protein)

4 oz. lean ground turkey

1 large onion, chopped

1 large garlic clove, minced

1 tablespoon chili powder

1 teaspoon ground cumin

2 teaspoons dried basil

1 teaspoon dried oregano

½ teaspoon salt or to taste

4 cups chopped tomatoes

1 (8-oz.) can tomato sauce

1 cup water

2 (15-oz.) cans black soybeans, drained and rinsed

Hot pepper sauce to taste

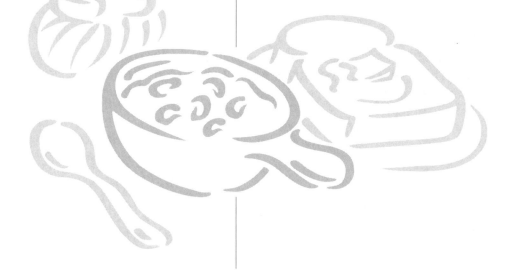

Add 1 cup boiling water to TSP in a medium bowl. Stir and let stand 10 minutes.

Cook turkey, onion and garlic in a large nonstick saucepan over medium heat, stirring to break up turkey, until turkey is no longer pink. Stir in rehydrated TSP, chili powder, cumin, basil, oregano and salt.

Add tomatoes, tomato sauce, water and soybeans. Cover and simmer, stirring occasionally, until onion is tender, about 20 minutes. Season with hot sauce to taste.

❋ Makes about 6 servings.

❋ 1 serving contains:
Cal 257	Prot 26g	Carb 22g
Fat 10g	Chol 16mg	Sodium 405mg

Variation
If black soybeans are not available, substitute canned or cooked dried black beans.

Vegetarian Chili

This is a good introduction to tempeh if you haven't had it before. The miso lends additional flavor that blends well with the vegetables.

2 teaspoons olive oil

1 cup chopped onion

1 large garlic clove, minced

½ cup chopped red bell pepper

½ cup chopped celery

1 (8-oz.) package soy tempeh, thawed if frozen

4 cups chopped tomatoes

1 cup water

1 (15-oz.) can cannellini or navy beans, drained and rinsed

1 tablespoon chili powder

1 teaspoon dried oregano

1 tablespoon red miso dissolved in ¼ cup hot water

Heat oil in a large nonstick saucepan over medium heat. Add onion, garlic, bell pepper and celery and cook, stirring occasionally, until softened, 5 to 8 minutes.

Crumble tempeh and add to vegetables. Stir in tomatoes, water, beans, chili powder and oregano. Cover and simmer, stirring occasionally, until onion is tender, about 20 minutes. Stir in miso mixture and heat until hot.

❊ Makes 4 servings.

❊ 1 serving contains:
Cal 285   Prot 19g   Carb 40g
Fat 8g   Chol 0mg   Sodium 187mg

salads

SOME OF MY FAVORITE SALADS HAVE BEEN made even better by the addition of soy. I now make a habit of adding soy in some form, whether it's cooked or roasted soybeans, soynuts or one of the creamy tofu dressings. For example, Two-Bean & Corn Salad showcases canned soybeans and creates one of the prettiest salads you've ever made. Pasta & Green Soybean Salad is also a feast for the eye as well as the taste buds.

Before using canned black or yellow beans in salads, drain them in a strainer and rinse well. Green soybeans are available frozen and they too are very easy to use. Cook the frozen green soybeans, cool them quickly, and—if in the pods—shell them before using. Cooking takes only a few minutes.

Crumbled, steamed tempeh and tofu are other soy products that can be used in salads too.

Because soy products are high in good-quality protein, almost all of the salads can be served as a main dish or as part of a salad buffet.

White Bean & Tofu Salad

Red onion and green pepper bring crispness to this wholesome salad. Serve it as part of a salad buffet for a lunch or light supper. Accompany with hot whole-wheat rolls or bread sticks.

¼ cup extra-virgin olive oil

2 tablespoons fresh lemon juice

2 tablespoons seasoned rice vinegar

1 tablespoon Dijon mustard

1 garlic clove, minced

2 tablespoons grated lemon zest

2 cups cooked or canned cannellini or navy beans, drained and rinsed

¼ cup chopped red onion

1 green bell pepper, finely chopped

8 oz. firm tofu, drained and cut into ½-inch cubes

Lettuce leaves

Chopped tomatoes

Whisk together olive oil, lemon juice, vinegar, mustard, garlic and lemon zest in a medium nonreactive bowl.

Stir in beans, onion, and bell pepper until coated. Gently stir in tofu. Cover and refrigerate 30 minutes, stirring occasionally.

Line 2 plates with lettuce leaves. Spoon salad over lettuce. Sprinkle chopped tomatoes over salad.

❁ Makes 2 main-dish servings.

❁ 1 serving contains:
Cal 497   Prot 25g   Carb 46g
Fat 25g   Chol 0mg   Sodium 148mg

Dilled Potato Salad

Everyone loves potato salad—a barbecue or picnic wouldn't be complete without it. This will become a favorite.

Cook potatoes in boiling salted water until tender, 15 to 20 minutes. Drain potatoes and transfer to a bowl. Sprinkle with rice vinegar and toss to combine. Cool potatoes to room temperature.

Stir in remaining ingredients. Refrigerate about 30 minutes for flavors to blend.

❀ Makes about 6 servings.

❀ 1 serving contains:

Cal 185	Prot 5g	Carb 42g
Fat 0.6g	Chol 0mg	Sodium 215mg

2 lb. russet potatoes, peeled and cut into small cubes

3 tablespoons seasoned rice vinegar or to taste

3 celery stalks, chopped

½ cup chopped sweet pickles

½ cup chopped onion

2 tablespoons chopped fresh parsley

1-½ teaspoons chopped fresh dill or ½ teaspoon dried

½ cup Creamy Dressing (page 46)

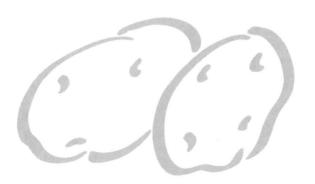

Tuna Salad–Stuffed Tomatoes

When vine-ripened tomatoes are at their peak, offer this as part of a perfect summer luncheon. Serve with a crunchy roll and iced tea.

1 (6-oz.) can water-packed tuna, drained

1 tablespoon fresh lemon juice

½ cup finely chopped celery

½ cup finely chopped red bell pepper

2 teaspoons minced fresh tarragon or ½ teaspoon dried

Freshly ground black pepper

About ¼ cup Creamy Dressing (page 46)

2 large tomatoes

Lettuce leaves

Minced green onions, including tops

Combine tuna, lemon juice, celery, bell pepper, tarragon, black pepper and dressing in a medium bowl. Cover and refrigerate.

Remove cores from tomatoes. Starting at the cored end and cutting almost through to the base, make three deep slices in each tomato to create 6 wedges. Line 2 plates with lettuce leaves. Place a tomato on each plate and open tomatoes to form a nest. Divide tuna salad among tomatoes. Sprinkle with green onions.

❈ Makes 2 main-dish servings.

❈ 1 serving contains:
| Cal 151 | Prot 25g | Carb 10g |
| Fat 2g | Chol 25mg | Sodium 407mg |

Pasta and Green Soybean Salad
see page 40

Toasted-Pecan and Mushroom Burger
see page 51

Crab Louie

Serve this classic dish for lunch or a light dinner. It's ideal for warm weather—no cooking is required for this elegant entrée.

Prepare dressing; set aside. Arrange salad greens in 2 large shallow bowls. Divide tomatoes, celery, carrots, crabmeat and onion rings between bowls.

Serve lemon wedges and dressing separately.

❋ Makes 2 main-dish servings.

❋ 1 serving contains:
Cal 236	Prot 30g	Carb 24g
Fat 3g	Chol 101mg	Sodium 602mg

Louie Dressing, (page 36)

About 4 cups mixed salad greens

2 medium tomatoes, chopped

2 celery stalks, cut crosswise into thin slices

2 small carrots, cut into thin strips

8 oz. crabmeat

6 or 8 small red onion rings

Lemon wedges

Louie Dressing

This dressing is also excellent as a dip for boiled shrimp or as a topping on grilled fish, such as salmon or sea bass.

½ cup Creamy
Dressing (page
46)

2 tablespoons
buttermilk or
plain,
unsweetened
soy milk

1 tablespoon fresh
lemon juice

2 tablespoons
chili sauce
or salsa

2 tablespoons
minced green
onion, including
tops

Whisk together all ingredients in a small bowl.

❋ Makes approximately ½ cup.

❋ 2 tablespoons contain:
Cal 24	Prot 2g	Carb 4g
Fat 0.5g	Chol 0mg	Sodium 177mg

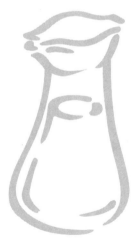

Two-Bean & Corn Salad

For best flavor, allow this salad to stand at room temperature about 30 minutes before serving. Taste the salad for seasoning and adjust, if needed.

Combine soybeans, corn, bell peppers and tomatoes in a medium bowl.

Whisk together vinegar, olive oil and garlic in a small bowl. Pour dressing over salad and toss to combine. Cover and refrigerate 2 hours or overnight, stirring occasionally.

❋ Makes 6 to 8 servings.

❋ 1 serving contains:
Cal 286	Prot 20g	Carb 30g
Fat 17g	Chol 0mg	Sodium 250mg

Variation

Southwestern Bean & Corn Salad: Add 1 minced serrano chile, ¼ cup finely chopped fresh cilantro and ½ teaspoon ground mild dried chile to the dressing.

1 (15-oz.) can yellow soybeans, drained and rinsed

1 (15-oz.) can black soybeans, drained and rinsed

2 cups cooked fresh or frozen whole-kernel corn, drained

1 cup finely chopped red bell pepper

1 cup finely chopped green bell pepper

3 medium Roma tomatoes, finely chopped

6 tablespoons seasoned rice vinegar

¼ cup extra-virgin olive oil

2 large garlic cloves, minced

Chicken, Baked Tofu & Noodle Salad
with Sesame Dressing

Baked tofu is found in the refrigerator section of your market. It's available plain or with a variety of seasonings.

Sesame Dressing
  (opposite page)

1 (6-oz.) package
  baked tofu, cut
  crosswise into
  thin strips

1 boneless, skinless
  chicken breast,
  cooked and cut
  into thin strips

1 cup jicama strips

1 red bell pepper, cut
  into thin strips

1 large carrot, cut
  into thin strips

1 medium zucchini,
  cut into thin strips

6 oz. buckwheat
  noodles, cooked
  according to
  package directions
  and drained

¼ cup minced green
  onions, including
  tops

¼ cup roasted soynuts

Prepare dressing; set aside. Combine tofu, chicken, jicama, bell pepper, carrot and zucchini in a medium bowl. Add about 2 tablespoons of dressing and toss to combine.

Place noodles in another bowl. Add about 2 tablespoons of dressing and toss to combine. Divide noodles among 4 plates. Top noodles with chicken-vegetable mixture. Sprinkle with green onions and roasted soynuts. Drizzle with remaining dressing.

❋ Makes 4 main-dish servings.

❋ 1 serving contains:
  Cal 250   Prot 23g   Carb 22g
  Fat 9g   Chol 18mg   Sodium 97mg

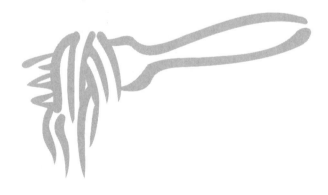

Sesame Dressing

Sesame oil has a more pronounced flavor than corn or canola oils. Look for it in your supermarket or Asian market.

Whisk together all ingredients in a small bowl.

❊ Makes about ½ cup.

❊ 2 tablespoons contain:
Cal 36	Prot 1g	Carb 1g
Fat 3g	Chol 0mg	Sodium 148mg

¼ cup seasoned rice vinegar

¼ cup fat-free, reduced-sodium chicken broth

1 tablespoon reduced-sodium soy sauce

1 tablespoon sesame oil

1 garlic clove, minced

Dash of hot pepper sauce

Pasta & Green Soybean Salad

Create a festive salad with Mediterranean flavors. Frozen green soybeans are sometimes called sweet beans. *They are available in the frozen-food section of natural-food stores.*

8 oz. small pasta shells, cooked according to package directions and drained

½ (16-oz.) package frozen green soybeans, cooked according to package directions and drained (see Note below)

1 red bell pepper, finely chopped

¼ cup finely chopped onion

¼ cup crumbled feta cheese

¼ cup chopped ripe Greek olives (optional)

¼ cup fat-free, reduced-sodium chicken broth

3 tablespoons white wine vinegar

2 tablespoons extra-virgin olive oil

1 tablespoon Dijon mustard

1 garlic clove, minced

2 tablespoons finely chopped fresh parsley

1 tablespoon finely chopped fresh basil or 1 teaspoon dried

1 teaspoon finely chopped oregano or ¼ teaspoon dried

Freshly ground black pepper to taste

Combine pasta, soybeans, bell pepper, onion, feta cheese and olives, if using, in a large bowl.

Whisk together chicken broth, vinegar, olive oil, mustard, garlic, herbs and pepper in a small bowl. Pour over pasta mixture and toss to combine. Cover and refrigerate at least 2 hours or overnight, tossing occasionally.

❄ Makes 6 to 8 servings.

❄ 1 serving contains:
| Cal 201 | Prot 8g | Carb 19g |
| Fat 11g | Chol 4mg | Sodium 290mg |

Note: If packaged, shelled green soybeans are not available in your area, check Asian markets for frozen green soybeans in the pods, called *edamamé*. Cook according to package directions, cool, shell and use as above. One pound of green soybeans in the pods yields 1-½ cups (8 oz.) after shelling.

Fried Tofu with Tossed Greens

The spicy coating flavors the tofu, but isn't as hot as the amounts would make you suspect. Everyone asks for more tofu!

1 (16-oz.) package extra-firm tofu, well drained

¼ cup all-purpose flour

1-½ teaspoons dried thyme

½ teaspoon cayenne pepper or to taste

½ teaspoon salt

½ teaspoon freshly ground black pepper

About ¼ cup olive oil

1 garlic clove, slivered

About 8 cups salad greens

Buttermilk Dressing (opposite page)

1 cup cherry tomatoes, cut in half if large

1 green bell pepper, cut into rings

Cut tofu into bite-size pieces and pat dry with paper towels. Combine flour, thyme, cayenne pepper, salt and pepper in a shallow dish and coat tofu with flour mixture.

Heat oil and garlic in a medium skillet over medium heat. Discard garlic when it browns. Add tofu in batches and cook until browned, about 3 minutes. Drain tofu on paper towels.

Toss salad greens and tomatoes with dressing. Divide salad among 4 salad plates. Top with bell pepper, cherry tomatoes and tofu.

✿ Makes 4 servings.

✿ 1 serving contains:

Cal 377	Prot 24g	Carb 23g
Fat 24g	Chol 0mg	Sodium 390mg

Variation

Spicy Tofu Wrap: Wrap the fried tofu, some chopped cabbage, cilantro and the dressing in warm whole-wheat tortillas for a great sandwich.

Buttermilk Dressing

Buttermilk dressing is especially good tossed with crisp mixed salad greens and sprinkled with roasted soynuts.

Whisk together all ingredients in a small bowl.

❄ Makes about ¾ cup.

❄ 2 tablespoons contain:
Cal 13	Prot 1g	Carb 1g
Fat 0.3g	Chol 0mg	Sodium 47mg

½ cup Creamy Dressing (page 46)

¼ cup buttermilk

1 tablespoon fresh lemon juice

¼ teaspoon sugar

1 teaspoon chopped fresh thyme, or ¼ teaspoon dried

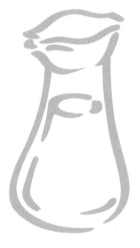

Curried Tempeh & Fruit Salad

An eye-catching salad that's a tangy treat for the palate.

1 (8-oz.) package tempeh, thawed if frozen

¼ cup Creamy Dressing (page 46)

¼ cup chopped chutney

1 teaspoon curry powder

Dash of hot pepper sauce

1 Granny Smith apple, unpeeled, chopped and tossed with 1 tablespoon fresh lemon juice

2 celery stalks, sliced crosswise

¼ cup raisins

Lettuce leaves

Cut tempeh into 1-inch cubes. Steam tempeh in a steamer basket over boiling water 20 minutes. Remove from steamer and cool.

Combine dressing, chutney, curry powder and hot pepper sauce in a small bowl. Combine apple, celery and raisins in a medium bowl. Add chutney dressing and tempeh and gently mix until combined.

Line 4 salad plates with lettuce leaves. Spoon salad over lettuce.

❈ Makes 4 servings.

❈ 1 serving contains:
Cal 198   Prot 12g   Carb 31g
Fat 5g   Chol 0mg   Sodium 88mg

Apple-Cabbage Slaw

Apple adds a nice juiciness to the slaw, and the vibrant colors make this an attractive addition to your menu.

Combine cabbage, carrot, bell peppers and apple with juice in a serving bowl. Add dressing and toss to coat. Cover and refrigerate 30 minutes before serving.

❀ Makes 6 servings.

❀ 1 serving contains:
| Cal 46 | Prot 2g | Carb 10g |
| Fat 0.6g | Chol 0mg | Sodium 58mg |

2 cups shredded cabbage

1 large carrot, shredded

½ cup finely chopped red bell pepper

½ cup finely chopped green bell pepper

1 Gala apple, unpeeled, finely chopped and tossed with 2 tablespoons fresh lemon juice

Buttermilk Dressing (page 43)

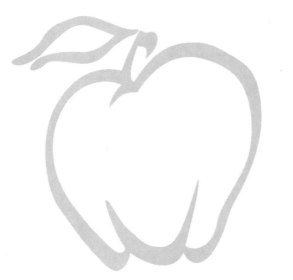

Creamy Dressing

Use this instead of mayonnaise in potato or other salads. If you don't tell, no one will know the difference. Nutritious Creamy Dressing has about half the fat of regular mayonnaise—plus healthful soy protein and no cholesterol.

1 cup (8 oz.) firm
   silken tofu, well
   drained

1 tablespoon
   Dijon mustard

2 tablespoons
   white-wine
   vinegar

Salt and pepper
   to taste

Process tofu in a food processor or blender until smooth. Add remaining ingredients and process to combine.

✻ Makes 1 cup.

✻ 1 tablespoon contains:
Cal 6	Prot 1g	Carb 0g
Fat 0.2g	Chol 0mg	Sodium 33mg

Variation

Herbed Creamy Dressing: Add 2 to 4 tablespoons of your favorite minced fresh or dried herbs.

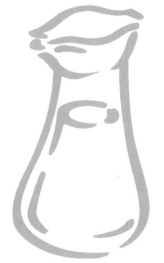

Blue Cheese Dressing

Serve with romaine lettuce or other sturdy salad greens.

Stir together all ingredients in a small bowl. Cover and refrigerate about 1 hour to enable flavors to blend.

❋ Makes about 1 cup.

❋ 2 tablespoons contain:
Cal 12	Prot 1g	Carb 0g
Fat 0.7g	Chol 2mg	Sodium 47mg

Variation

Easy Blue Cheese Dip: Omit buttermilk. Combine remaining ingredients, including garlic.

½ cup Creamy Dressing (page 46)

¼ cup buttermilk

¼ cup crumbled blue cheese

1 garlic clove (optional), minced

Freshly ground black pepper

Avocado Dressing

This creamy, refreshing avocado dressing is excellent with seafood or vegetable salads. The oil in avocados is mostly monounsaturated, similar to canola and olive oils.

½ small avocado

1 tablespoon capers

1 tablespoon fresh lemon juice

1 tablespoon minced fresh parsley

½ cup Creamy Dressing (page 46)

1 small garlic clove, minced

Freshly ground black pepper

Process avocado and capers in a food processor until almost smooth. Add remaining ingredients, process to combine and transfer to a small bowl. Cover and refrigerate about 1 hour to enable flavors to blend.

❋ Makes about 1 cup.

❋ 2 tablespoons contain:
| Cal 14 | Prot 0g | Carb 1g |
| Fat 1g | Chol 0mg | Sodium 24mg |

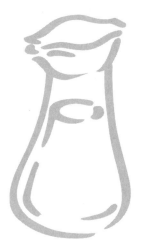

main dishes

BESIDES THE USUAL TOFU, CONSIDER experimenting with other products to add soy to your main dishes. Options include tempeh, TSP (textured soy protein), whole soybeans in different forms, meat alternatives made from soy protein and soy cheeses.

The following recipes offer new ways to incorporate soy into your diet easily. Many of these recipes will sound familiar and contain chicken, beef or seafood in addition to soy. Chicken & Tempeh Curry will introduce you to one of the delicious combinations possible.

As you became more comfortable with soy products, you may want to create your own recipes and increase the amount of soy you use, while decreasing the amount of meat.

Chicken & Tempeh Curry

*The combination of chicken and tempeh is better than either one alone.
I prefer using fresh rather than frozen spinach in this recipe.*

*Serve this curry with cooked basmati rice. Sprinkle raisins and pistachio
nuts over the curry if you like.*

8 oz. boneless,
skinless chicken
breast

1 (8-oz.) package
soy tempeh

1 tablespoon
olive oil

1 medium onion,
quartered and
sliced lengthwise

1 large garlic clove,
minced

8 oz. (about 6)
small white
potatoes,
quartered

8 oz. baby carrots

2 celery stalks,
sliced crosswise

1-½ lb. fresh
tomatoes,
chopped

1 tablespoon curry
powder

½ teaspoon ground
cinnamon

¾ teaspoon salt

3 cups packed
baby spinach

Cut chicken and tempeh into bite-size pieces; set
aside. Heat oil in a large pan over medium heat. Add
onion and garlic and cook until softened. Remove
with a slotted spoon. Add chicken and cook, stirring
occasionally until browned. Add tempeh and cook,
stirring occasionally, about 5 minutes.

Add potatoes, carrots, celery, tomatoes, curry powder,
cinnamon and salt. Cover and simmer, stirring
occasionally, until vegetables are tender, about
30 minutes. Stir in spinach and cook 5 minutes more.

❀ Makes 4 to 6 servings.

❀ 1 serving contains:

Cal 373	Prot 27g	Carb 40g
Fat 14g	Chol 36mg	Sodium 528mg

Toasted-Pecan & Mushroom Burgers

Toasted pecans and mushrooms add a meatlike texture and flavor to this burger. Serve on whole-wheat English muffins with tomato, spinach leaves and red onion slices. Top with cheese if desired.

Preheat oven to 400F (205C). Crumble tofu with a fork. Place between paper towels to drain.

Heat the olive oil in a skillet over medium heat. Add onion, carrot and garlic and cook, stirring occasionally, until vegetables begin to soften, about 5 minutes. Add mushrooms; cook, stirring occasionally, until most of moisture evaporates. Add sherry; cook, stirring occasionally, until moisture evaporates. Cool slightly.

In a food processor, combine tofu, vegetable mixture, ketchup, mustard, thyme, salt, hot pepper sauce and pecans. Pulse just until mixed. Using about $1/3$ cup of mixture for each, shape into 4 patties.

Arrange patties on a baking sheet that has been sprayed with nonstick cooking spray. Lightly spray patties with cooking spray. Bake until lightly browned on bottom, 15 to 20 minutes.

❋ Makes 4 burgers.

❋ 1 burger contains:

Cal 285	Prot 7g	Carb 13g
Fat 25g	Chol 0mg	Sodium 495mg

1 cup (8 oz.) extra-firm low-fat tofu, drained

1 tablespoon olive oil

½ cup finely chopped onion

½ cup shredded carrot

1 garlic clove, minced

1 cup finely chopped mushrooms

1 tablespoon sherry

2 tablespoons ketchup

1 tablespoon Dijon mustard

½ teaspoon dried thyme

½ teaspoon salt

Dash of hot pepper sauce

1 cup pecans, toasted (see Note, page 110) and finely chopped

Bulgur-Vegetable Burgers

A tender vegetarian burger with flavorful spices. The addition of egg white contributes good-quality protein and helps hold together this delicate burger. Serve in whole-wheat pita pockets with tomato, lettuce and onion.

1 cup (8 oz.) extra-firm low-fat tofu, drained

1 tablespoon olive oil

½ cup finely chopped onion

½ cup finely chopped celery

½ cup shredded zucchini

1 garlic clove, minced

2 tablespoons finely chopped Niçoise olives

½ cup softened bulgur (see Note, next page)

1 egg white

1 tablespoon fresh lime juice

1 teaspoon ground mild chile

½ teaspoon ground cumin

½ teaspoon dried oregano

½ teaspoon salt

Dash of hot pepper sauce

¼ cup plain wheat germ

Preheat oven to 400F (205C). Crumble tofu with a fork. Place between paper towels to drain.

Heat the olive oil in a skillet over medium heat. Add onion, celery, zucchini and garlic and cook, stirring occasionally, until vegetables are softened, about 10 minutes. Cool slightly.

In a food processor, combine tofu, vegetable mixture, olives, bulgur, egg white, lime juice, ground chile, cumin, oregano, salt and hot pepper sauce. Pulse just until mixed. Using about $1/3$ cup of mixture for each, shape into 4 patties. Pour wheat germ into a shallow dish. Coat both sides of patties with wheat germ, patting in wheat germ slightly.

Arrange patties on a baking sheet that has been sprayed with nonstick cooking spray. Lightly spray patties with cooking spray. Bake until lightly browned on bottom, 15 to 20 minutes.

❋ Makes 4 burgers.

❋ 1 burger contains:

Cal 120	Prot 8g	Carb 12g
Fat 5g	Chol 0mg	Sodium 370mg

Note: Bulgur triples in volume when hot water is added. To make ½ cup softened bulgur, pour about $1/3$ cup hot water over 3 tablespoons dried bulgur; let stand 15 to 20 minutes. Squeeze out excess water.

Tomato-Herb Pasta Sauce

A medley of vegetables adds interest to this versatile sauce. The recipe can be halved and the remaining Gimme Lean!™ frozen to use in another recipe. Or make the full recipe and freeze any extra pasta sauce for up to 1 month. This is especially good with penne pasta.

2 teaspoons olive oil

1-½ cups chopped onion

1 celery stalk, chopped

1 garlic clove, minced

1 (14-oz.) package Gimme Lean!™ soy product

1 cup shredded carrot

1 cup sliced mushrooms

1 (28-oz.) can chopped tomatoes

1 (15-oz.) can tomato sauce

2 teaspoons dried basil

1 teaspoon dried oregano

Hot pepper sauce

½ teaspoon salt or to taste

Heat 1 teaspoon olive oil in a large nonstick saucepan over medium-low heat. Add onion, celery and garlic and cook, stirring occasionally, until softened, about 5 minutes. Add remaining 1 teaspoon olive oil and Gimme Lean! and cook over medium heat until browned, cutting up Gimme Lean! until it resembles ground meat.

Stir in carrot and mushrooms. Add tomatoes with juice, tomato sauce, basil, oregano and a dash of hot pepper sauce. Simmer about 20 minutes for flavors to blend. Season with salt.

❀ Makes 8 cups.

❀ 1 serving contains:

Cal 127	Prot 10g	Carb 19g
Fat 2g	Chol 0mg	Sodium 835mg

Chicken & Roasted Vegetable Pasta

A hearty casserole for family or friends that reflects the flavors of Italy.

Preheat oven to 350F (175C). Spray a nonstick roasting pan with nonstick cooking spray. Arrange eggplant and garlic in prepared pan. Roast about 30 minutes or until soft and remove. Cool vegetables, peel and coarsely chop (keeping vegetables separate).

Cook penne according to package directions until tender to the bite, and drain. Place in a large bowl. Combine garlic, tofu, vinegar, olive oil, basil, salt and black pepper in a food processor and process until blended. Add chicken broth and process until combined. Add eggplant, chicken, tomatoes and capers to pasta. Spoon sauce over mixture and stir to combine.

Transfer mixture to a 2-quart casserole dish. (If you assemble this dish ahead, cover and refrigerate. Increase baking time by about 10 minutes.) Bake about 30 minutes or until hot and bubbly. Sprinkle with cheese and bake about 5 minutes more or until cheese melts.

❋ Makes 6 servings.

❋ 1 serving contains:

Cal 218	Prot 18g	Carb 21g
Fat 7g	Chol 37mg	Sodium 375mg

1 (1-lb.) eggplant

4 cloves garlic (unpeeled)

8 oz. penne pasta

1 cup (8 oz.) silken tofu, drained

3 tablespoons balsamic vinegar

1 tablespoon olive oil

2 tablespoons minced fresh basil, or 1 teaspoon dried

½ teaspoon salt or to taste

Coarsely ground black pepper to taste

½ cup chicken broth

8 oz. cooked chicken, cut into bite-size pieces

4 Roma tomatoes, chopped

1 tablespoon capers, drained

¼ cup freshly grated Parmesan cheese

Stuffed Bell Peppers

Currants and pine nuts supply subtle flavor to an old favorite. Look for short, broad bell peppers with even bottoms. The stuffing could also be used for green chiles.

4 medium green, red or yellow bell peppers

1 (8-oz.) package soy tempeh, crumbled

¼ cup pine nuts, toasted (see Note, page 110)

½ cup currants

4 green onions, minced

2 garlic cloves, minced

¼ cup chopped parsley

1 teaspoon ground cinnamon

½ teaspoon ground allspice

1 (8-oz.) can tomato sauce

2 tablespoons fresh lemon juice

Preheat oven to 350F (175C). Spray a nonstick baking pan with nonstick cooking spray. Slice the stem ends off each bell pepper and reserve. Discard cores and seeds. Set bell peppers aside.

Combine all remaining ingredients in a medium bowl. Stuff tempeh mixture into bell peppers. Arrange stuffed bell peppers in prepared pan and cover with reserved bell pepper tops. Add about ¼ cup water to pan and cover with foil. Bake about 60 minutes or until bell peppers are tender.

❋ Makes 4 servings.

❋ 1 serving contains:
Cal 235	Prot 16g	Carb 23g
Fat 11g	Chol 0mg	Sodium 350mg

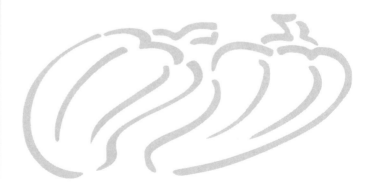

Sloppy Joes

My version of this traditional dish. Serve over baked potatoes or whole-wheat hamburger buns. This is an easy way to add tempeh to your menus.

Crumble tempeh into a medium saucepan. Add remaining ingredients and bring to a boil. Reduce heat, cover and simmer over low heat 20 minutes or until vegetables and tempeh are tender, add water if mixture becomes too thick.

❊ Makes 2 or 3 servings.

❊ 1 serving contains:

Cal 269	Prot 17g	Carb 42g
Fat 6g	Chol 0mg	Sodium 985mg

1 (8-oz.) package 5-grain tempeh, thawed if frozen

1 (8-oz.) can tomato sauce

½ cup ketchup

2 tablespoons light brown sugar

1 cup finely chopped onion

1 cup finely chopped celery

½ cup chopped green bell pepper

1 garlic clove, minced

1 teaspoon dry mustard

1 teaspoon dried thyme

Dash of hot pepper sauce or to taste

Water, if needed

Eggplant Rollatina with Marinara Sauce

Eggplant is one of my favorite vegetables, so I am always trying it in new ways. Individual rolls, easily served, make an ideal buffet entrée. Tofu blended with mozzarella seems like another layer of cheese.

2 cups purchased tomato pasta sauce or Easy Marinara Sauce (opposite page)

1 large eggplant

Olive oil spray

½ (16-oz.) package extra-firm tofu, drained

1 tablespoon dried basil

1 teaspoon dried oregano

1 garlic clove, minced

1-½ cups (6 oz.) shredded part-skim mozzarella

EASY MARINARA SAUCE:

1 teaspoon olive oil

1 medium onion, finely chopped

1 celery stalk, finely chopped

1 garlic clove, minced

1 (15-oz.) can crushed tomatoes

1 teaspoon dried basil

½ teaspoon dried oregano

Freshly ground black pepper

Prepare Marinara Sauce and keep warm or heat purchased sauce.

Preheat broiler. Remove stem end and slice eggplant lengthwise into 8 to 10 thin slices. Spray both sides with olive oil spray and place in 1 layer on a nonstick baking sheet. Broil about 5 minutes or until soft, turning once.

Slice tofu crosswise into 8 to 10 equal slices and place on paper towels. Spray a nonstick baking sheet with olive oil spray. Broil tofu about 5 minutes or until very lightly browned on top.

Preheat oven to 400F (205C). Spray a nonstick baking pan with olive oil spray. Lay tofu slices over eggplant slices and sprinkle with herbs and garlic. Sprinkle with 1 cup of the cheese. Roll, starting at a short end, to enclose cheese and place seam-side down in prepared pan, securing rolls with wooden picks. Spoon sauce over eggplant and bake about 30 minutes. Sprinkle with remaining cheese and bake 10 minutes or until cheese melts and sauce is bubbly. Remove wooden picks before serving.

Easy Marinara Sauce

Heat oil in a nonstick saucepan over medium-low heat. Add onion, celery and garlic and cook, stirring occasionally, until vegetables are softened, about 5 minutes. Add tomatoes, herbs and pepper, cover and simmer about 10 minutes or until vegetables are tender. Makes about 2 cups.

❀ Makes 6 servings.

❀ 1 serving contains:
Cal 180   Prot 15g   Carb 11g
Fat 9g   Chol 15mg   Sodium 278mg

Savory Salmon Crepes

Stacked crepes are easy to assemble and look attractive when cut into wedges. A fresh dill garnish and a tossed salad make this festive enough for a special luncheon.

CREPES:

½ cup all-purpose flour

¼ cup buckwheat flour

1-¼ cups fat-free plain, unsweetened soy milk

2 egg whites

2 tablespoons soft margarine, melted, or vegetable oil

¼ teaspoon salt

FILLING:

1 (12.3-oz.) package extra-firm low-fat silken tofu, drained

1 tablespoon soy sauce

Dash of hot pepper sauce or to taste

1 (6-oz.) can boneless salmon, drained

1 cup cooked chopped broccoli

½ cup cooked chopped leeks

1 tablespoon snipped fresh dill or 1 teaspoon dried dill weed

Salt and freshly ground black pepper

TO ASSEMBLE:

½ cup shredded Monterey jack cheese

Make crepe batter: Combine all ingredients in a blender or food processor and process until smooth. Pour batter into a large glass measuring cup or pitcher. Cover and refrigerate 1 hour.

Make filling: Add tofu, soy sauce and hot pepper sauce to a food processor and process until smooth. Add salmon and pulse to evenly chop. Stir in broccoli, leeks, dill, salt and pepper.

To cook crepes, heat a well-seasoned or nonstick 7-inch crepe pan or skillet over medium. Spray with nonstick cooking spray. Stir batter. Pour about 3 tablespoons of batter into center of pan, tilting pan quickly so batter covers bottom completely. Cook until bottom of crepe is brown. Turn crepe and cook until bottom of crepe is light brown. Remove crepe to a plate and continue making crepes with remaining batter. Put a sheet of waxed paper between each crepe. Makes about 12 crepes.

To assemble, preheat oven to 425F (220C). Spray a baking sheet with nonstick cooking spray. Place 2 crepes on baking sheet. Spread 1/12 of filling on each crepe. Repeat with remaining crepes and filling to make 2 stacks of 6 crepes each. Sprinkle top with cheese. Bake 20 minutes or until filling is hot and cheese is melted.

❋ Makes 6 servings.

❋ 1 serving contains:
   Cal 113   Prot 8g   Carb 8g
   Fat 6g   Chol 9mg   Sodium 113mg

Black Bean, Beef & Tofu Loaf

Meat loaf takes on a new look and flavor. An egg white helps hold together this loaf. Make sure the tofu is well drained before using.

1 cup (8 oz.) extra-firm tofu, drained

1 (15-oz.) can black soybeans, drained and rinsed

1 egg white

1 small onion, chopped

¼ cup ketchup

1 tablespoon Worcestershire sauce

Freshly ground black pepper

2 tablespoons minced fresh parsley

12 oz. extra-lean ground beef

Preheat oven to 350F (175C). Spray a nonstick 9 x 5-inch loaf pan with nonstick cooking spray. Combine tofu and beans in a food processor and pulse until puréed. Add egg white, onion, ketchup and seasoning and pulse just until combined. Mix in beef with your hands until evenly distributed.

Transfer beef mixture to prepared pan and smooth top. Bake about 55 minutes or until top is browned and an instant-read thermometer inserted in center registers 165F (75C). Let cool in pan 10 minutes. Pour off any liquid that remains. Cut into slices.

✽ Makes about 6 servings.

✽ 1 serving contains:
Cal 260	Prot 26g	Carb 11g
Fat 12g	Chol 56mg	Sodium 224mg

New-Fashioned Meat Loaf

A colorful salsa topping adds extra appeal to this dish. I find that using an electric mixer is the easiest way to blend the rehydrated TSP with the ground beef and other ingredients.

Preheat oven to 350F (175C). Spray a nonstick 9 x 5-inch loaf pan with nonstick cooking spray. Add boiling water to TSP in a large bowl. Stir and let stand 10 minutes.

Using an electric mixer, beat in remaining ingredients, except salsa, until evenly combined.

Transfer beef mixture to prepared pan and smooth top. Bake about 50 minutes or until top is browned and an instant-read thermometer inserted in center registers 165F (75C). Let cool in pan 10 minutes. Cut into slices. Serve with salsa, if desired.

❋ Makes 4 to 6 servings.

❋ 1 serving contains:
Cal 426   Prot 46g   Carb 20g
Fat 19g   Chol 112mg   Sodium 715mg

1 cup boiling water

⅞ cup TSP (textured soy protein)

1 lb. lean ground beef

½ cup rolled oats

1 (8-oz.) can tomato sauce

1 small onion, finely chopped

1 celery stalk, finely chopped

2 garlic cloves, minced

2 teaspoons dried thyme

½ teaspoon salt or to taste

Freshly ground black pepper

Papaya-Avocado Salsa (page 64) (optional)

Papaya-Avocado Salsa

Lime juice enhances the flavors of both of these tropical fruits. It also helps preserve the delicate colors.

1 small avocado, peeled and cut into ¼-inch cubes

1 small papaya, peeled and cut into ¼-inch cubes

2 tablespoons finely chopped red onion

1 tablespoon grated lime zest

2 tablespoons fresh lime juice

1 teaspoon sugar

¼ teaspoon ground mild red chile

Combine all ingredients in a medium bowl.

❀ Makes about 3 cups.

❀ 2 tablespoons contain:
Cal 20　　Prot 0g　　Carb 2g
Fat 1g　　Chol 0mg　　Sodium 2mg

Note: Select a ripe avocado that yields easily when pressed but is not too soft, indicating that it is overripe. A ripe papaya is slightly soft when pressed, and the skin is yellow.

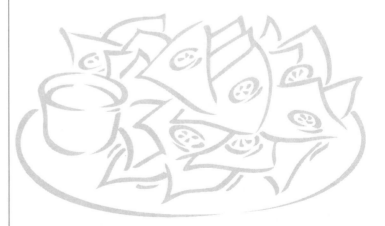

Beef & Bean Wraps

Try the different flavors of tortillas or special wraps that are now available, such as blue corn, whole-wheat or tomato. I prefer a hot green salsa with this, but choose your own favorite.

Combine beef, bell peppers, onion, garlic and salt in a large skillet over medium heat. Cook, stirring to break up beef, until beef is no longer pink. Stir in soybeans, tomato and hot pepper sauce and heat, stirring occasionally, until hot.

Spoon beef mixture in center of each tortilla. Top with salsa, if using. Fold one side of tortilla over filling, then fold in remaining sides. Serve warm.

❋ Makes 4 servings.

❋ 1 serving contains:
| Cal 349 | Prot 28g | Carb 30g |
| Fat 13g | Chol 56mg | Sodium 471mg |

Note: Tortillas warm quickly in a microwave oven. Or wrap in foil and heat in a 350F (175C) oven about 10 minutes.

8 oz. extra-lean ground beef

½ red bell pepper, chopped

½ green bell pepper, chopped

1 cup chopped red onion

1 garlic clove, minced

½ teaspoon salt or to taste

1 (15-oz.) can black soybeans, drained and rinsed

1 medium tomato, chopped

Dash of hot pepper sauce

4 (about 7-inch) flour tortillas, warmed (see Note)

Salsa (optional)

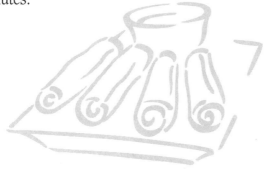

Onion-Cheese Strudel

Serve warm slices of flaky filo, stuffed with cheese and herbs, with a tossed green salad for a light lunch or supper.

1 tablespoon soft margarine

3 large sweet onions, thinly sliced

1 garlic clove, minced

2 tablespoons finely chopped sun-dried tomatoes

1 teaspoon dried thyme

1 teaspoon dried marjoram

¼ teaspoon salt or to taste

Coarsely ground black pepper

1 cup (8 oz.) extra-firm low-fat tofu, drained

4 oz. blue cheese, crumbled

2 tablespoons fresh lemon juice

10 to 12 filo pastry sheets

About ¼ cup soft margarine, melted

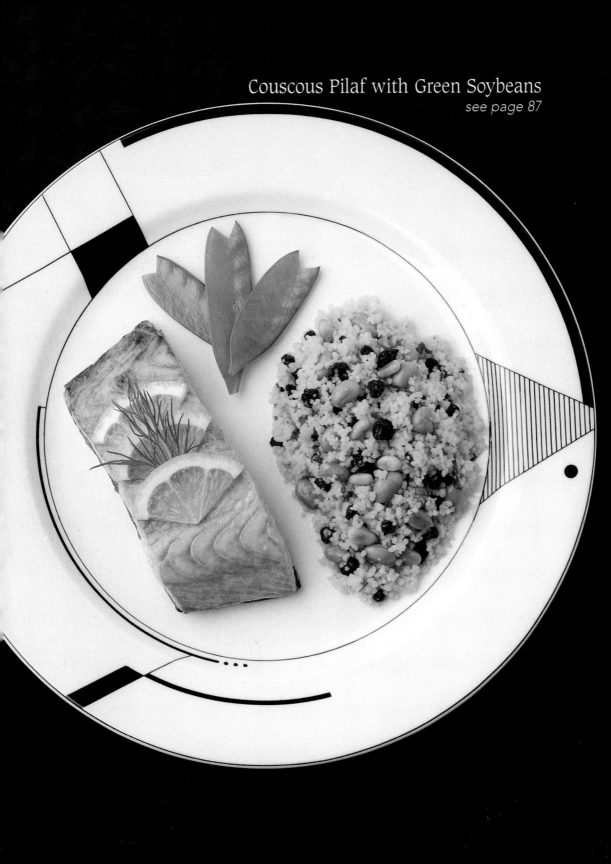

Couscous Pilaf with Green Soybeans
see page 87

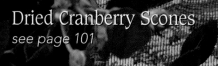

Dried Cranberry Scones
see page 101

Preheat oven to 375F (190C). Spray a baking sheet with nonstick cooking spray. Melt margarine in a large skillet over low heat. Add onions and garlic, cover and cook, stirring occasionally, until onions are very soft, about 15 minutes. Stir in tomatoes, thyme, marjoram, salt and pepper. Cool slightly.

Process tofu in a food processor until smooth. Stir in blue cheese and lemon juice. Stir tofu mixture into vegetable mixture in skillet.

Place 1 filo sheet on a work surface and cover remaining pastry with plastic wrap to prevent drying. Brush filo sheet very lightly with melted margarine and top with another sheet of pastry. Continue with remaining pastry sheets and margarine.

Spoon filling over pastry, leaving a 2-inch border on all sides. Fold in ends and roll to enclose filling. Place on prepared baking sheet and brush top with margarine. Bake about 30 minutes or until golden brown.

To serve, cut crosswise into about 2-½-inch pieces with a serrated knife. Serve warm.

❋ Makes about 8 servings.

❋ 1 serving contains:

| Cal 251 | Prot 10g | Carb 20g |
| Fat 15g | Chol 11mg | Sodium 468mg |

Stacked Bean Quesadillas

When black soybeans are blended in the food processor, the texture is similar to refried black beans. The bean mixture can be used as a filling for wraps or enchiladas or used almost anywhere refried beans are used. Serve the wedges with your favorite salsa and slices of avocado.

1 teaspoon olive oil

½ cup chopped green bell pepper

2 tablespoons minced onion

1 garlic clove, minced

1 (15-oz.) can black soybeans, drained

½ cup (4 oz.) soft tofu, drained

2 Roma tomatoes, chopped

1 tablespoon mild ground chile

Hot pepper sauce to taste

6 (about 7-inch) whole-wheat tortillas

4 oz. goat cheese, crumbled

½ cup chopped fresh cilantro

Preheat oven to 375F (190C). Spray a nonstick baking sheet with nonstick cooking spray. Heat olive oil in a nonstick skillet over medium-low heat. Add bell pepper, onion and garlic and cook, stirring, until softened, about 5 minutes.

Process beans, tofu and tomatoes in a food processor or blender until puréed. Add vegetables and ground chile. Season with hot pepper sauce.

Arrange 2 tortillas on prepared baking sheet. Spread each tortilla with ⅓ of the bean mixture. Sprinkle each tortilla with ⅓ of the goat cheese and ⅓ of the cilantro. Top each with a tortilla. Repeat with bean mixture and goat cheese and remaining tortillas. Bake about 15 minutes or until cheese is melted and bean mixture is hot. Cut into wedges.

❊ Makes about 6 servings.

❊ 1 serving contains:

Cal 225	Prot 14g	Carb 23g
Fat 9g	Chol 9mg	Sodium 228mg

Schnitzel mit Tofu

My rendition of a German classic. Serve as an entrée with steamed fresh asparagus and boiled red potatoes.

Slice tofu crosswise into 8 equal slices and place on paper towels. Trim ham and cheese to fit on tofu slices with about ½-inch border on all sides. Top half the tofu slices with half the cheese, then the ham. Spread ham with mustard and top with remaining cheese. Top with remaining tofu slices.

Combine flour, thyme and pepper in a shallow bowl. Carefully coat both sides of tofu stack with flour mixture. Heat oil in a large nonstick skillet. Add tofu and cook until browned on bottom. Carefully turn and cook until browned on other side and cheese melts, about 5 minutes total cooking time. Serve warm.

❈ Makes 4 servings.

❈ 1 serving contains:
Cal 141	Prot 11g	Carb 13g
Fat 5g	Chol 13mg	Sodium 502mg

Variations

1. Top ham slices with fresh sage leaves.

2. Bake in a preheated 400F (205C) oven about 10 minutes or until cheese melts. Top with a pasta sauce and bake until hot.

½ (16-oz.) package extra-firm tofu, drained

4 thin slices cooked ham

4 thin slices provolone-style soy cheese

2 teaspoons honey mustard

½ cup all-purpose flour

2 teaspoons dried thyme

Freshly ground black pepper

2 tablespoons olive oil

Tuna Balls & Mustard-Chutney Sauce

Surprise your family with this unusual mix of flavors.

1 (6-oz.) water-pack tuna, drained

2 tablespoons dried breadcrumbs

2 egg whites, lightly beaten

1 teaspoon dry mustard

¼ cup minced green onions

1 teaspoon dried thyme

Dash of cayenne

½ (16-oz.) extra-firm frozen tofu, pressed and shredded (see Note, opposite)

Cooked rice, to serve

MUSTARD-CHUTNEY SAUCE:

¼ cup finely chopped mango chutney

¼ cup Creamy Dressing (page 46)

1 tablespoon honey mustard

About ¼ cup apple juice

Combine all ingredients except rice and sauce in a medium bowl. Cover and refrigerate 30 minutes until mixture becomes somewhat firm.

Preheat oven to 400F (205C). Spray a nonstick baking sheet with nonstick cooking spray. Using 2 tablespoons of mixture for each, shape into balls.

Arrange balls on prepared baking sheet. Bake 18 to 20 minutes or until balls are browned. Serve warm with Mustard-Chutney Sauce over rice.

❈ Makes 4 (3 tuna balls each) servings.

❈ 1 serving contains:
| Cal 132 | Prot 17g | Carb 12g |
| Fat 1g | Chol 13mg | Sodium 399mg |

Mustard-Chutney Sauce

Combine chutney, dressing and mustard in a small bowl. Stir in enough apple juice to make desired consistency. Cover and refrigerate until served.

❈ Makes about ¾ cup.

Note: Because tofu is perishable, every tofu package has a "use by" date. If you buy more than you need, you may freeze the extra tofu in its package. (An exception is silken tofu packed in aseptic packages.) After freezing and thawing, squeeze the tofu to remove all of the liquid. The texture will be sponge-like, and like a sponge, the defrosted tofu will absorb seasoning and liquids easily.

Use frozen tofu when the moisture content of regular tofu would add too much moisture.

Taco Noodle Casserole

Don't tell the kids there is no beef in their favorite casserole. Serve with steamed broccoli and sliced tomatoes.

1 (4-oz.) package soy taco filling

2 cups (8 oz.) pennette or other pasta

¼ cup all-purpose flour

2 cups unsweetened, plain soy milk

1 small onion, finely chopped

1 cup finely chopped celery

1 red bell pepper, chopped

2 teaspoons dried oregano

1 teaspoon salt or to taste

Freshly ground white pepper to taste

Dash of hot pepper sauce

1 cup (4 oz.) shredded Monterey jack cheese

Preheat oven to 350F (175C). Spray a shallow 2-quart casserole dish with nonstick cooking spray. Prepare taco filling according to package directions and set aside. Cook pasta according to package directions until tender but firm to the bite and drain. Combine taco filling and pasta in prepared casserole dish.

Combine flour and a little soy milk in a medium saucepan over medium heat. Stir in remaining milk and vegetables and cook, stirring, until thickened, about 5 minutes. Add oregano, salt, white pepper, hot pepper sauce and cheese and cook, stirring, until cheese melts.

Pour sauce over mixture in casserole dish and stir to combine. Bake about 30 minutes or until bubbly and top is browned.

✽ Makes about 6 servings.

✽ 1 serving contains:

Cal 228	Prot 19g	Carb 25g
Fat 8g	Chol 17mg	Sodium 488mg

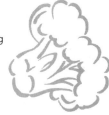

Chiles Rellenos

Mild green chiles are stuffed with provolone-style soy cheese.

Preheat oven to 350F (175C). Spray an
8-inch-square baking pan with cooking spray.
Arrange chiles in prepared pan and stuff with cheese.

Beat egg whites with salt until stiff but not dry. Fold
in flour and tofu. Pour tofu mixture over chiles. Bake
about 30 minutes or until topping is lightly browned.
Serve hot.

❋ Makes 4 servings.

❋ 1 serving contains:
Cal 187	Prot 17g	Carb 12g
Fat 9g	Chol 0mg	Sodium 393mg

5 large mild fresh
or canned green
chiles, roasted,
peeled and
seeds removed
(see Note,
page 2)

5 slices (²/₃ oz. each)
provolone-style
soy cheese

3 egg whites

½ teaspoon salt

2 tablespoons all-
purpose flour

1 cup (8 oz.) soft
tofu, drained
and pureed

Dilled Salmon Patties

Doubly delicious when you top these patties with Louie Dressing, page 36. Because all the water is pressed from the thawed tofu, it is easy to form patties or meatballs.

1 (16-oz.) package
firm tofu, frozen

1 (14.75-oz.) can
red salmon,
drained

¼ cup minced
onion

¼ cup chopped
fresh dill

2 tablespoons
chopped fresh
parsley

2 tablespoons fresh
lemon juice

¼ cup low-fat
mayonnaise

Thaw tofu in package in cold water. Remove tofu from package and drain. Press water from tofu and tear into pieces. Place tofu and salmon in a food processor; process until chopped. Add onion, dill, parsley, lemon juice and mayonnaise; process until combined. Form into patties, using ¼ cup of mixture for each cake.

Spray a nonstick large skillet with cooking spray and heat over medium heat. Add patties and cook until browned on both sides, turning once, about 8 minutes total cooking time.

❀ Makes about 8 patties.

❀ 1 serving contains:
   Cal 183   Prot 20g   Carb 4g
   Fat 10g   Chol 25mg   Sodium 328mg

Tempeh Teriyaki

Asian flavors abound in each bite. Serve with steamed rice and fresh green beans.

Cut tempeh crosswise into 2 equal pieces. Cut each half diagonally into 2 triangles, making a total of 4 triangles. Steam tempeh in a steamer basket over boiling water 20 minutes.

Meanwhile, combine remaining ingredients in a small saucepan. Stir over medium heat until honey dissolves; set aside.

Preheat oven to 350F (175C). Spray a shallow baking dish large enough to hold tempeh triangles in a single layer with cooking spray. Arrange tempeh in prepared baking dish. Pour tamari mixture over tempeh.

Bake 20 minutes, basting occasionally with sauce, until sauce is absorbed and tempeh is browned.

❋ Makes 2 servings.

❋ 1 serving contains:
| Cal 411 | Prot 27g | Carb 44g |
| Fat 15g | Chol 0mg | Sodium 1631mg |

1 (8-oz.) package tempeh

¼ cup tamari

2 tablespoons honey

2 tablespoons sherry

1 teaspoon olive oil

2 garlic cloves, minced

1 tablespoon minced ginger root

2 green onions, minced

2 tablespoons sesame seeds

Dash of hot pepper sauce

Variation
Recipe can be doubled.

side dishes

MOST OF US LIKE TO TRY NEW SIDE DISHES to accompany our favorite entrées. Here you'll find grains and vegetables combined with various soy products. Tofu, soy milk and the different forms of the soybeans themselves are easy to incorporate into flavorful side dishes. Because soy products contain protein, you reap the benefit of adding good-quality protein to your diet.

This chapter also contains basic recipes for cooking dried soybeans and green soybeans. One of my favorite recipes, for Roasted Soybeans, is included here. Roasted soybeans are delightfully versatile: They can be eaten as a snack or used to top casseroles and salads. You will probably discover your own favorite uses for these tasty, crunchy beans.

Basic Cooked Dried Soybeans

Dried soybeans take almost twice as long to cook as other dried beans. For this reason, cooking in a slow cooker is a good option. The freshness of the soybeans will determine the cooking time; older soybeans take longer to cook. Soybeans that have been stored for more than two years may not get completely tender, even after cooking for a long time. As with all dried beans, do not salt the soybeans until they are tender, near the end of their cooking time, because salt toughens beans.

1 lb. (about 2 cups) dried soybeans

Sort through soybeans and discard broken beans and debris. Place soybeans in a strainer and rinse. Add soybeans to a large saucepan or bowl and cover with about 4 inches of cold water; soak overnight. Drain beans and rinse.

Add soaked soybeans and 6 cups water to a large saucepan. Boil 5 minutes. Reduce heat, cover and simmer 3 to 4 hours or until soybeans are tender.

❀ Makes 5 to 6 cups.

❀ 1 cup contains:
Cal 377   Prot 33g   Carb 27g
Fat 18g   Chol 0mg   Sodium 2mg

Variations

Slow Cooker Method: Soak soybeans as above and drain. Add soybeans and about 4 cups water to a slow cooker. Cook on HIGH 6 to 8 hours or until soybeans are tender.

Pressure Cooker Method: Soak soybeans as above and drain. Add soybeans, about 5 cups water and 1 tablespoon vegetable oil to a pressure cooker, filling the pressure cooker no more than half full. Bring to HIGH pressure and cook 35 to 45 minutes. Let pressure return to normal. Or follow directions for your pressure cooker.

Green Shelled Soybeans

Sometimes called sweet beans, *frozen green shelled soybeans are not quite as easy to find as dried soybeans. That should change in the near future, because their popularity is growing. Green soybeans are harvested when they are about 80% mature, so they cook quickly—in about 10 minutes.*

1 (16-oz.) package
    frozen green
    soybeans

¼ teaspoon salt or
    to taste

Cook soybeans according to package directions. Serve hot as a vegetable or add to recipes.

❋ Makes 5 or 6 servings.

❋ 1 serving contains:
    Cal 100   Prot 9g   Carb 11g
    Fat 5g   Chol 0mg   Sodium 144mg

Variation

Rice and Beans: Toss cooked soybeans with 1 cup cooked brown rice, minced green onion and ½ teaspoon dried thyme. Heat until hot. Sprinkle with grated part-skim mozzarella cheese, if desired.

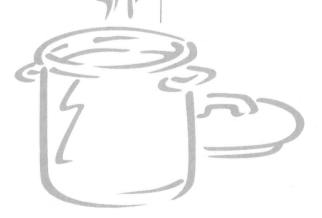

Green Soybeans in Pods

Also called edamamé, *green soybeans are available in the freezer section in markets where Japanese foods are sold, as well as in some natural-food markets. Boiled and salted soybeans in the pods are sometimes offered as a starter in sushi restaurants (in the same way that salsa and chips may be offered in Mexican restaurants).*

Add soybeans and salt to a large saucepan of boiling water. Boil 10 minutes. Drain and cool. Remove beans and discard pods.

Serve soybeans as a green vegetable or use in recipes.

❀ Makes 1-½ cups.

❀ ½ cup contains:
| Cal 90 | Prot 9g | Carb 3g |
| Fat 5g | Chol 0mg | Sodium 363mg |

1 (16-oz.) package frozen green soybeans in pods

½ teaspoon salt

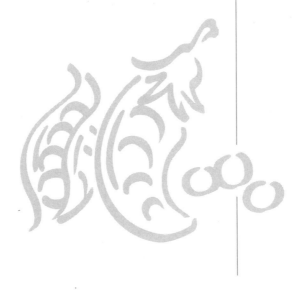

Roasted Soybeans

Roasted soybeans, called soynuts, *are available commercially, but you can make your own.*

1 cup dried
   soybeans

¼ teaspoon salt or
   to taste

Sort through soybeans and discard broken beans and debris. Place soybeans in a strainer and rinse. Add soybeans to a large saucepan or bowl and cover with about 4 inches of cold water and soak overnight. Rinse beans and drain well.

Preheat oven to 300F (150C). Lightly spray a nonstick baking sheet with olive oil. Spread soaked soybeans on baking sheet. Spray with olive oil spray. Bake, stirring every 15 minutes, about 1 hour or until soybeans are crunchy and lightly browned. Sprinkle with salt.

❋ Makes about 1 cup.

❋ 1 tablespoon contains:

Cal 51	Prot 4g	Carb 4g
Fat 2g	Chol 0mg	Sodium 33mg

Garlic & Herb Mashed Potatoes

Perfect for someone who is lactose intolerant; no milk is used in these potatoes. The tofu blends in so well that no one will know it's there unless you say so.

Bring potatoes to a boil in water to cover; cover and simmer until tender, about 20 minutes.

Meanwhile, melt margarine or butter in a skillet over medium heat. Add garlic and herbs; cook, stirring occasionally, until mixture bubbles and is fragrant, about 2 minutes. Set aside.

Drain potatoes and mash. Beat in tofu, herb mixture, salt and pepper to taste. Keep warm over very low heat until served.

❁ Makes 4 servings.

❁ 1 serving contains:

Cal 205	Prot 6g	Carb 38g
Fat 3g	Chol 8mg	Sodium 572mg

1-½ lbs. russet potatoes, peeled and cut into pieces

1 tablespoon soft margarine or butter

2 large garlic cloves, minced

¼ cup chopped fresh parsley

1 teaspoon chopped fresh oregano

½ teaspoon chopped fresh thyme

¾ cup (6 oz.) soft silken tofu

1 teaspoon salt

Freshly ground black pepper

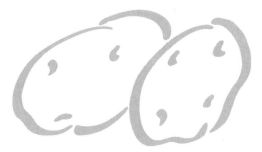

Creamed Spinach Casserole

You can prepare this flavorful dish year-round by substituting well-drained, cooked, frozen spinach for the fresh spinach.

1 lb. fresh spinach

½ cup (4 oz.) soft silken tofu

½ cup unsweetened, plain soy milk

2 tablespoons all-purpose flour

1 onion, very finely chopped

1 red bell pepper, chopped

2 garlic cloves, minced

¼ cup chopped sun-dried tomatoes

1 teaspoon dried savory

2 to 4 tablespoons slivered almonds

Preheat oven to 350F (175C). Spray a 2-quart casserole dish with nonstick cooking spray. Wash spinach, remove large stems and coarsely chop. Cook spinach in the water clinging to the leaves in a large saucepan over medium heat until wilted. Drain spinach; set aside.

Combine tofu, soy milk and flour in a food processor and pulse until smooth. Stir in spinach, onion, bell pepper, garlic, tomatoes and savory. Transfer mixture to prepared casserole dish. Cover and bake 20 minutes. Uncover, sprinkle with almonds and bake 15 minutes more or until bubbly and almonds are browned.

❁ Makes 4 servings.

❁ 1 serving contains:
Cal 104	Prot 8g	Carb 13g
Fat 4g	Chol 0mg	Sodium 184mg

Mushroom & Asparagus Bake

One of my springtime favorites is fresh asparagus. Here I combine it with mushrooms and top it off with a smooth sauce. Crimini are small, brown, button mushrooms. Substitute with white button mushrooms if crimini are not available.

Wipe mushrooms and cut into thick slices. Cook asparagus in boiling water until crisp-tender and drain well.

Preheat oven to 350F (175C). Spray a shallow 2-quart casserole dish with nonstick cooking spray. Spread asparagus in prepared casserole dish. Lay mushrooms over asparagus.

Beat together soy milk, flour and onion in a medium saucepan. Cook over medium heat, stirring, until thickened and bubbly. Season with salt and pepper to taste. Pour sauce over vegetables. Sprinkle with breadcrumbs. Bake about 30 minutes or until bubbly and top is browned.

✳ Makes 4 servings.

✳ 1 serving contains:
Cal 110   Prot 6g   Carb 20g
Fat 2g   Chol 0mg   Sodium 649mg

8 oz. small crimini mushrooms

1 lb. fresh asparagus, trimmed

½ cup plain, unsweetened soy milk

1 tablespoon all-purpose flour

2 tablespoons minced onion

Salt and freshly ground pepper

½ cup seasoned breadcrumbs

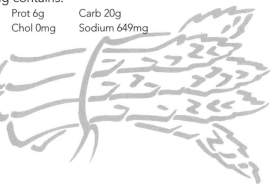

Bulgur Casserole

Soy grits are coarsely ground. This dish is reminiscent of a hearty Spanish rice.

½ cup bulgur

½ cup soy grits

2 cups hot water

1 celery stalk, finely chopped

1 small onion, finely chopped

½ cup chopped Roma tomatoes

½ cup finely chopped green bell pepper

Preheat oven to 350F (175C). Combine bulgur and soy grits in a 2-quart casserole dish. Stir in hot water and let stand 15 minutes or until most of water is absorbed.

Stir in celery, onion, tomatoes and bell pepper. Cover and bake about 30 minutes. Remove cover and bake about 20 minutes more, or until vegetables are tender.

✽ Makes 6 servings.

✽ 1 serving contains:

Cal 114	Prot 7g	Carb 16g
Fat 4g	Chol 0mg	Sodium 11mg

Couscous Pilaf with Green Soybeans

Saffron, an exotic spice from the crocus flower, adds distinctive flavor and golden color. Couscous, available in most supermarkets, is a precooked pasta that cooks in minutes.

Bring water, saffron and salt to a boil in a large saucepan. Stir in couscous, currants and soybeans, and cover. Remove from heat and let stand 5 minutes.

Stir in mint, parsley and pine nuts. Serve warm or at room temperature.

❀ Makes about 6 servings.

❀ 1 serving contains:

Cal 184	Prot 10g	Carb 29g
Fat 4g	Chol 0mg	Sodium 198mg

1-½ cups water

1/8 teaspoon saffron threads, crushed

½ teaspoon salt or to taste

1-½ cups couscous

½ cup currants

1 cup cooked green soybeans (page 80)

2 tablespoons chopped fresh mint

2 tablespoons chopped fresh parsley

2 tablespoons pine nuts, toasted (see Note, page 110)

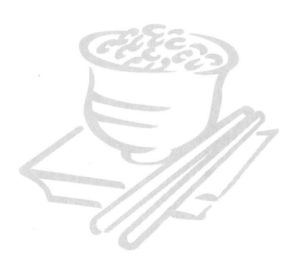

Twice-Baked Potatoes

Always a favorite, these are made with soy yogurt and soy cheese, so they contain no cholesterol, yet have lots of flavor.

2 large baking
   potatoes

½ cup soy yogurt

1 teaspoon Dijon
   mustard

4 oz. (1 cup) finely
   chopped
   Cheddar-style
   soy cheese

¼ cup minced
   chives

½ teaspoon salt
   or to taste

Freshly ground
   black pepper

Preheat oven to 400F (205C). Scrub potatoes and place in a small baking pan. Bake about 1 hour or until soft.

Cool potatoes slightly. Cut potatoes in half and scoop out interiors into a bowl, leaving a thin wall of potato within the potato skin. Add yogurt and mustard to potato pulp and beat until smooth. Stir in cheese, chives, salt and pepper.

Return potato mixture to potato shells. Place filled potatoes in a baking dish. Bake about 20 minutes or until hot and tops are browned.

❋ Makes 4 servings.

❋ 1 serving contains:
| Cal 118 | Prot 4g | Carb 22g |
| Fat 2g | Chol 0mg | Sodium 38mg |

Variation

Bake 2 or 3 large unpeeled garlic cloves with potatoes until soft, about 15 minutes. Press cloves out of garlic heads into a small bowl and mash with a fork. Add garlic to potato mixture with chives.

Easy Spicy Cheese Sauce

Spoon cheese sauce over steamed broccoli or cauliflower, or use it as a topping for baked potatoes. The sauce becomes very thick as it cools; to thin, reheat with a little additional soy milk.

Combine soy cheese and soy milk in a small saucepan over low heat and cook, stirring constantly, until cheese melts, about 5 minutes.

❋ Makes ¾ cup.

❋ 2 tablespoons contain:
Cal 11	Prot 1g	Carb 1g
Fat 0.5g	Chol 0mg	Sodium 20mg

3 oz. jalapeño-flavored soy cheese, chopped

½ cup unsweetened, plain soy milk

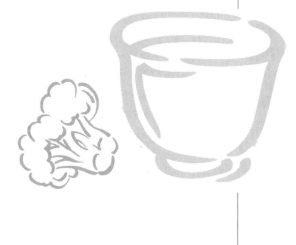

Green Soybeans, Corn and Tomatoes

A colorful side dish that could also be a vegetarian entrée for two. Serve with Light Cornbread (page 93) and a mixed green salad.

1 teaspoon extra-virgin olive oil

1 cup chopped onion

1 cup frozen green soybeans

½ cup water

1 (11-oz.) can whole-kernel corn, drained

2 cups chopped fresh or canned tomatoes

½ teaspoon chopped fresh sage

Salt and freshly ground black pepper, to taste

Heat oil in a medium nonstick saucepan over medium heat. Add onion and sauté, stirring occasionally, until softened, about 5 minutes. Add soybeans and water. Cover and simmer 5 minutes.

Add corn, tomatoes, sage, salt and pepper. Cover and simmer until vegetables are tender, about 5 minutes. Serve hot.

❀ Makes 4 servings.

❀ 1 serving contains:
Cal 207   Prot 12g   Carb 30g
Fat 7g   Chol 0mg   Sodium 458mg

Tip: *If you haven't purchased new nonstick cookware recently, you might want to consider buying a new saucepan or skillet. The nonstick surfaces have improved and are better than ever. Just a spritz of nonstick cooking spray or 1 teaspoon of olive oil for flavor is all the fat needed with these new surfaces. After buying a new sauté pan recently, I went back for matching saucepans.*

breads

AN UNEXPECTED BONUS OF USING SOY FLOUR or tofu in bread and other baked goods is that the breads do not seem to become stale as quickly. They retain moisture—they even become moister the day *after* baking. For this reason it's wise to freeze these breads unless you plan to use them within two or three days.

If you want to experiment with soy flour in your own recipes, replace 2 tablespoons per cup of all-purpose flour with soy flour. If you like the results, keep going, and replace another tablespoon of flour with the soy flour the next time. Beware of adding too much soy flour; in this case, where soy flour is concerned, there *can* be too much of a good thing. Soy flour does not contain gluten, so if you use too much of it, your bread will be denser and won't rise as expected.

Double-Corn Muffins

Cream-style corn serves a dual purpose; it adds extra flavor and also contributes part of the liquid.

1-½ cups cornmeal

½ cup all-purpose flour

1 teaspoon sugar

1 tablespoon baking powder

1 teaspoon ground mild red chile

¼ teaspoon salt

1 (8-oz.) can cream-style corn

2 tablespoons vegetable oil

¾ cup (6 oz.) soft tofu, drained and puréed

¼ cup finely chopped green onions with tops

½ cup cubed jalapeño soy cheese (optional)

Preheat oven to 425F (220C). Spray 12 muffin cups with nonstick cooking spray.

Combine cornmeal, flour, sugar, baking powder, ground chile and salt in a medium bowl. Beat corn, oil and tofu in another bowl until combined. Stir tofu mixture into cornmeal mixture until just combined. Stir in onions and cheese, if using. Spoon batter into prepared muffin cups.

Bake 15 to 20 minutes or until tops spring back when lightly pressed.

Cool muffins in pan 10 minutes before serving or cooling completely on a wire rack.

❋ Makes 18 muffins.

❋ 1 muffin contains:
Cal 76   Prot 2g   Carb 13g
Fat 2g   Chol 0mg   Sodium 158mg

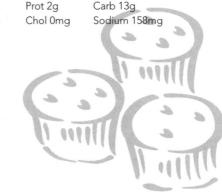

Light Cornbread

This is a very light cornbread. I prefer to bake it in a well-seasoned cast-iron skillet or cornstick pan, which I preheat in the oven before adding the batter. This gives a crisp crust and also reduces the baking time.

Preheat oven to 375F (190C). Spray a medium cast-iron skillet or 8-inch baking pan with nonstick cooking spray. Preheat the skillet, if using.

Combine cornmeal, bread flour, soy flour, baking powder, sugar and salt in a medium bowl. Beat together egg, soy milk and oil in a small bowl. Stir egg mixture into dry ingredients just until combined.

Pour batter into prepared skillet. Bake 15 to 20 minutes or until top springs back when lightly pressed and the bottom and edges are browned. Cut into wedges and serve warm.

❋ Makes 4 or 5 servings.

❋ 1 serving contains:
Cal 206   Prot 7g   Carb 32g
Fat 6g   Chol 47mg Sodium 340mg

1 cup cornmeal

¼ cup bread flour

2 tablespoons defatted soy flour

2 teaspoons baking powder

1 teaspoon sugar

⅛ teaspoon salt

1 egg or 2 egg whites

½ cup unsweetened, plain soy milk

1 tablespoon extra-virgin olive oil

Cream Biscuits

Don't let the name fool you; these are made with soy cream cheese and milk but taste like they were made with cream. Together they make tender, delicious biscuits. They taste great with strawberry preserves.

1 cup self-rising flour (see Tip, below)

3 tablespoons soy cream cheese

About ⅓ cup plain, unsweetened soy milk

Preheat oven to 425F (220C). Spray a small baking sheet with nonstick cooking spray.

Add flour to a medium bowl. Cut in cream cheese until mixture is crumbly. Stir in enough milk to make a soft dough. Turn out dough on a lightly floured surface and knead 4 or 5 times. Pat out dough to a ½-inch thickness. Using a round 2-inch cutter, cut out rounds. Reroll scraps and cut into biscuits.

Arrange biscuits about 2 inches apart on prepared baking sheet. Bake about 8 minutes or until lightly browned on bottoms. Serve warm.

❀ Makes about 8 biscuits.

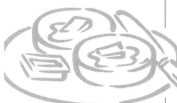

❀ 1 biscuit contains:

Cal 72	Prot 2g	Carb 12g
Fat 1g	Chol 3mg	Sodium 216mg

Tip: *I prefer to use soft-wheat self-rising flour, because it is low in gluten and makes biscuits even more tender. All-purpose self-rising flour works, too; be careful not to over-knead or the biscuits will be tough.*

Toasted Pecan & Currant Muffins

Toasted pecans accent the natural nutty flavor of soy flour.

Preheat oven to 425F (220C). Spray 9 muffin cups with nonstick cooking spray. Combine flours, baking powder, salt and cinnamon in a medium bowl. Beat egg, honey, soy milk and vanilla extract in another bowl until smooth. Stir egg mixture into flour mixture until just combined. Gently stir in pecans and currants.

Spoon batter into prepared muffin cups. Bake 15 to 20 minutes or until tops spring back when lightly pressed.

Cool muffins in pan 10 minutes before serving or cooling completely on a wire rack.

❋ Makes 9 muffins.

❋ 1 muffin contains:

Cal 120	Prot 3g	Carb 19g
Fat 4g	Chol 24mg	Sodium 186mg

1 cup all-purpose flour

2 tablespoons defatted soy flour

2 teaspoons baking powder

¼ teaspoon salt

1 teaspoon ground cinnamon

1 egg or 2 egg whites

3 tablespoons honey

½ cup fat-free vanilla soy milk

1 teaspoon pure vanilla extract

¼ cup chopped pecans, toasted (see Note, page 110)

¼ cup dried currants

Lemon Poppy-Seed Muffins

These tender muffins have a light, moist texture and fresh grated lemon adds to the delightful flavor. For variety, substitute orange juice and peel for the lemon.

1 cup all-purpose flour

½ cup white whole-wheat flour (see Note, opposite)

2 teaspoons baking powder

½ teaspoon baking soda

¼ teaspoon salt

1 cup soy yogurt

¼ cup honey

¼ cup soft margarine

¼ cup fresh lemon juice

1 tablespoon grated lemon zest

2 tablespoons poppy seeds

LEMON GLAZE (OPTIONAL):

¼ cup fresh lemon juice

¼ cup sugar

Preheat oven to 425F (220C). Spray 12 muffin cups with nonstick cooking spray. Combine flours, baking powder, baking soda and salt in a medium bowl. Beat yogurt, honey, margarine and lemon juice in another bowl until smooth. Stir yogurt mixture into flour mixture until just combined. Stir in lemon zest and poppy seeds.

Spoon batter into prepared muffin cups. Bake 15 to 20 minutes or until tops spring back when lightly pressed.

Make glaze, if using, and drizzle over muffins. Cool muffins in pan 10 minutes before serving or cooling completely on a wire rack.

✽ Makes 12 muffins.

✽ 1 muffin contains:
  Cal 133   Prot 3g   Carb 19g
  Fat 5g   Chol 0mg   Sodium 212mg

Lemon Glaze

Stir together lemon juice and sugar in a small bowl. Spoon over muffins in pan.

Note: White whole-wheat flour is available by mail from the King Arthur Flour Company and is also available at most Trader Joe's stores.

Cranberry–Pumpkin Muffins

Dried cranberries have become one of my favorite additions to muffins and other baked products. They also make great snacks.

2 cups all-purpose flour

¼ cup defatted soy flour

1 tablespoon baking powder

¼ teaspoon salt

2 teaspoons ground cinnamon

1 teaspoon ground allspice

¼ cup packed light brown sugar

1 cup canned or cooked puréed pumpkin

1 cup fat-free vanilla soy milk

2 tablespoons vegetable oil

1 cup dried cranberries

Preheat oven to 400F (205C). Spray 12 muffin cups with nonstick cooking spray. Stir together flours, baking powder, salt, cinnamon, allspice and sugar in a medium bowl.

Stir together pumpkin, soy milk and oil in another bowl. Stir pumpkin mixture into dry ingredients just until combined. Stir in cranberries.

Spoon batter into muffin cups, filling each cup ⅔ full. Bake about 20 minutes or until browned.

Cool muffins in pan 10 minutes before serving or cooling completely on a wire rack.

✼ Makes 12 muffins.

✼ 1 muffin contains:

Cal 169	Prot 4g	Carb 32g
Fat 3g	Chol 0mg	Sodium 172mg

Breakfast Wraps and
Papaya-Strawberry Smoothie
see pages 120 and 126

Creamy Cherry Parfait
see page 131

Fresh Apple Bread

If you like moist quick breads, you'll want to make this one often.

Preheat oven to 350F (175C). Spray a nonstick 9 x 5-inch loaf pan with nonstick cooking spray.

Beat together margarine, brown sugar, tofu, soy milk and vanilla in a medium bowl. Combine flour, cinnamon, cloves, baking soda, baking powder and salt in a small bowl. Add flour mixture to tofu mixture and beat until combined. Stir in apple with juice. Pour batter into prepared loaf pan.

Bake about 1 hour or until top springs back when lightly pressed. Cool in pan 10 minutes on a wire rack. Turn out of pan and allow to cool completely before slicing.

❋ Makes 1 loaf, about 9 slices.

❋ 1 slice contains:
Cal 207	Prot 4g	Carb 35g
Fat 6g	Chol 0mg	Sodium 283mg

¼ cup soft margarine

½ cup packed light brown sugar

½ cup (4 oz.) soft tofu, drained and puréed

½ cup fat-free vanilla soy milk

1 teaspoon pure vanilla extract

2 cups all-purpose flour

2 teaspoons ground cinnamon

½ teaspoon ground cloves

1 teaspoon baking soda

½ teaspoon baking powder

¼ teaspoon salt

1 cup shredded apple, tossed with 1 tablespoon fresh lemon juice

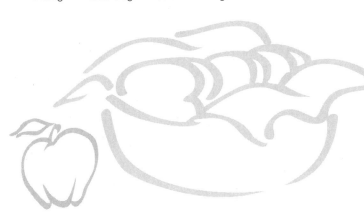

Double-Ginger Banana Bread

Rich ginger flavor permeates this moist banana bread. Serve in thin slices topped with cream cheese to rave reviews.

¾ cup packed light brown sugar

½ cup soft margarine

½ cup (4 oz.) tofu, drained and puréed

2 teaspoons pure vanilla extract

1 cup mashed ripe bananas (about 2 medium)

2 cups all-purpose flour

1 teaspoon baking soda

¼ teaspoon salt

1 teaspoon ground ginger

1 teaspoon ground allspice

2 tablespoons finely chopped candied ginger

½ cup chopped nuts (optional)

Preheat oven to 350F (175C). Spray a nonstick 9 x 5-inch loaf pan with nonstick cooking spray.

Beat brown sugar and margarine in a medium bowl until light and fluffy. Beat in tofu, vanilla and bananas until combined. Stir together flour, baking soda, salt, ground ginger and allspice in another bowl. Add flour mixture to banana mixture and stir just until combined. Stir in candied ginger and nuts, if using.

Spoon batter into prepared loaf pan. Bake about 45 minutes or until center springs back when lightly pressed. Cool in pan 10 minutes and turn out on a wire rack to finish cooling.

❁ Makes 1 loaf, 10 slices.

❁ 1 slice contains:

| Cal 250 | Prot 4g | Carb 38g |
| Fat 10g | Chol 0mg | Sodium 269mg |

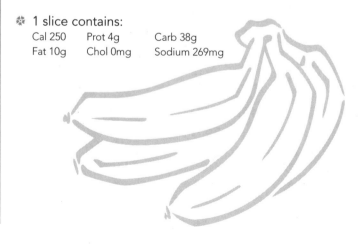

Dried Cranberry Scones

Serve these for tea or with your morning coffee. Unlike regular scones, these will still be moist on the second day because of the soy flour they contain.

Preheat oven to 400F (205C). Spray a nonstick baking sheet with nonstick cooking spray. Stir together flours, sugar, baking powder and salt in a medium bowl.

Stir in margarine until mixture forms crumbs. Stir in milk and almond extract to make a soft dough. Stir in cranberries or cherries and almonds, if using.

Turn out dough on a lightly floured board and knead lightly. Roll out dough to a 3/4-inch thickness. Cut into 12 triangles.

Place triangles on prepared pan. Bake 12 to 15 minutes or until browned. Serve warm.

❈ Makes about 12 scones.

❈ 1 scone contains:

Cal 157	Prot 4g	Carb 27g
Fat 4g	Chol 0mg	Sodium 201mg

2 cups all-purpose flour

¼ cup whole-wheat flour

¼ cup defatted soy flour

3 tablespoons sugar

1 tablespoon baking powder

¼ teaspoon salt

¼ cup soft margarine

²/₃ cup fat-free vanilla soy milk

1 teaspoon pure almond extract

½ cup chopped dried cranberries or cherries

¼ cup slivered almonds (optional)

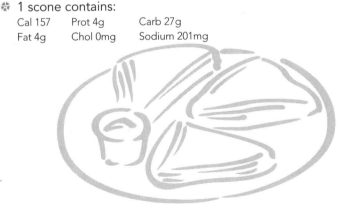

Spiced Fruit & Nut Yeast Bread

The sweetness here comes from the dried figs, golden raisins and honey. The spices and vanilla complement the lemon zest and add a wonderful aroma.

2 tablespoons margarine or butter

2 tablespoons honey

1 teaspoon salt

1 teaspoon ground cinnamon

¼ teaspoon ground cloves

1 teaspoon pure vanilla extract

1 tablespoon fresh lemon juice

Grated zest from 1 medium lemon

1 cup fat-free vanilla soy milk

1 egg

2-½ cups bread flour

¼ cup defatted soy flour

¾ cup white whole-wheat flour (see Note, page 97)

2 teaspoons active dry yeast

½ cup golden raisins

½ cup diced figs

½ cup chopped walnuts

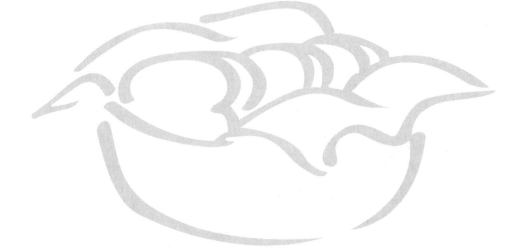

Add ingredients, except fruit and nuts, in order listed to a bread machine container. Set machine for "raisin bread." Add raisins, figs and walnuts at the beep. (If your machine doesn't have a raisin-bread setting, add the fruit and nuts during the middle-to-end of the second knead.) Check dough for consistency and add a tablespoon of water or bread flour as needed.

❋ Makes 1 large loaf, 12 slices.

❋ 1 slice contains:
Cal 229   Prot 8g   Carb 37g
Fat 7g   Chol 15mg   Sodium 205mg

Variation

To make without a bread machine: Dissolve the yeast in ¼ cup warm water in a large bowl. Let stand until foamy, about 5 minutes. Add margarine, honey, salt, cinnamon, cloves, vanilla, lemon juice and zest, soy milk and egg; beat until combined. Beat in soy flour and whole-wheat flour. Add enough of the bread flour to make a moderately stiff dough. Add raisins, figs and walnuts and stir until evenly distributed.

Turn out dough on a floured surface and knead until smooth. Place in a greased bowl and cover. Let rise in a warm place until doubled in size, about 2 hours. Punch down dough and shape into a loaf. Place in a greased 9 x 5-inch loaf pan. Cover and let rise until almost doubled in size, about 1 hour. Preheat oven to 350F (175C). Bake bread about 50 minutes or until browned and loaf sounds hollow when tapped on bottom. Cool on a wire rack before cutting.

Apricot & Currant Drop Scones

Drop scones need no rolling; just drop them onto the baking sheet. Make these when you are short on time.

1-½ cups all-purpose flour

¾ cup whole-wheat flour

1 tablespoon baking powder

¼ teaspoon salt

1 teaspoon ground cinnamon

¼ teaspoon ground ginger

¼ cup soft margarine

1-¼ cups fat-free vanilla soy milk

¼ cup pure maple syrup

2 teaspoons pure vanilla extract

¼ cup chopped dried apricots

¼ cup chopped dried currants

Preheat oven to 400F (205C). Spray a nonstick baking sheet with nonstick cooking spray. Stir together flours, baking powder, salt, cinnamon and ginger in a medium bowl.

Stir in margarine until mixture forms crumbs. Stir in milk, maple syrup and vanilla to make a very soft dough. Stir in apricots and currants.

Drop dough by about 2 tablespoons onto prepared baking sheet. Bake about 15 minutes or until browned. Serve warm.

❀ Makes 12 scones.

❀ 1 scone contains:

Cal 154	Prot 4g	Carb 25g
Fat 4g	Chol 0mg	Sodium 203mg

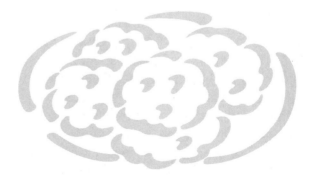

breakfast dishes

BREAKFAST, MY FAVORITE AND THE MOST important meal, is often the most neglected meal of the day. We feel that we don't have time or that many of the foods we like are on the "no" list. Fortunately, breakfast menus are easily enhanced with soy products. If you are cutting down on cholesterol and saturated fat, you can use tofu and defatted soy flour to replace all or part of the eggs in many dishes. For example, the Southwestern Egg Scramble uses both eggs and tofu, but in the pancakes and waffles all the eggs have been replaced.

Using TSP (textured soy protein) with ground pork to make your own sausage is another way to make your breakfast more healthful. Try the already seasoned and commercially packaged sausage substitutes in breakfast dishes.

So enjoy soy for breakfast and forget the guilt!

Blueberry Pancakes with Orange-Maple Syrup

Nutritious and delicious, maybe this is the true breakfast of champions. Two grains (wheat and oats) plus soy flour add fiber, protein, B vitamins and iron—a special way to start the day.

Orange-Maple Syrup (opposite page)

1-½ cups all-purpose flour

2 tablespoons defatted soy flour

2 tablespoons wheat germ

½ cup old-fashioned rolled oats

1 tablespoon baking powder

¼ teaspoon salt

2 cups fat-free vanilla soy milk

1 tablespoon honey

¼ cup (2 oz.) silken tofu, drained and puréed

2 tablespoons vegetable oil

1 teaspoon pure vanilla extract

1 cup fresh or thawed frozen blueberries

Make syrup and keep warm. Combine flours, wheat germ, oats, baking powder and salt in a medium bowl. Combine milk, honey, tofu, oil and vanilla in a small bowl. Stir milk mixture into flour mixture just until combined. Gently stir in blueberries.

Spray a nonstick griddle with nonstick cooking spray and place over medium heat. Using about ⅓ cup batter for each pancake, cook pancakes on hot griddle until bubbles form. Turn pancakes and cook until lightly browned on underside, about 2 minutes.

❃ Makes about 12 (5-inch) pancakes.

❃ 1 pancake and ¼ cup syrup contain:
Cal 216   Prot 5g   Carb 42g
Fat 4g   Chol 0mg   Sodium 178mg

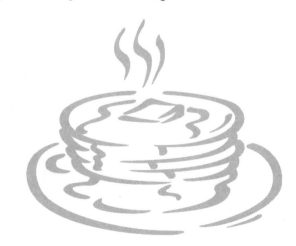

Orange-Maple Syrup

Oranges and orange juice add flavor and vitamin C. They also help decrease the sweetness of the syrup.

Stir together cornstarch and ¼ cup of the orange juice in a medium saucepan until smooth. Stir in remaining orange juice and maple syrup. Cook over low heat, stirring constantly, until thickened. Chop orange segments and add to syrup with zest. Serve warm.

❁ Makes about 3 cups.

❁ 2 tablespoons contains:

Cal 46	Prot 0g	Carb 12g
Fat 0g	Chol 0mg	Sodium 2mg

1-½ tablespoons cornstarch

1 cup fresh orange juice

1 cup pure maple syrup

1 medium orange, peeled and segmented

2 tablespoons grated orange zest

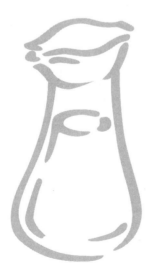

Whole-Wheat Pancakes with Double-Apricot Syrup

Perhaps these delicious pancakes should be called the "nuts and seeds" pancakes. Flax seed is a good source of omega-3 fatty acids and lignans—a phytochemical that may help prevent cancer. Store flax seed and flax seed oil in the refrigerator.

Double-Apricot Syrup (opposite page)

1-½ cups all-purpose flour

½ cup whole-wheat flour

1 tablespoon ground flax seed

1 tablespoon light brown sugar

1 tablespoon baking powder

¼ teaspoon salt

2-¼ cups fat-free vanilla soy milk

2 tablespoons vegetable oil

1 teaspoon pure vanilla extract

2 tablespoons sunflower kernels

2 teaspoons sesame seeds

Make syrup and keep warm. Combine flours, flax seed, sugar, baking powder and salt in a medium bowl. Combine soy milk, oil and vanilla in a small bowl. Stir milk mixture into flour mixture just until combined. Gently stir in seeds.

Spray a nonstick griddle with nonstick cooking spray and place over medium heat. Using about ⅓ cup batter for each pancake, cook pancakes on hot griddle until bubbles form. Turn pancakes and cook until lightly browned on underside, about 2 minutes.

❋ Makes about 12 (5-inch) pancakes.

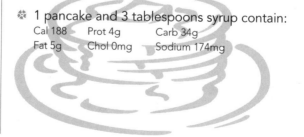

❋ 1 pancake and 3 tablespoons syrup contain:

Cal 188	Prot 4g	Carb 34g
Fat 5g	Chol 0mg	Sodium 174mg

Double-Apricot Syrup

Dried apricots are particularly versatile and can be used in sauces, baked goods and as a snack. Rich in beta carotene, apricots complement the flavors of many foods.

Combine apricot nectar, apricots, sugar and lemon juice in a medium saucepan. Cook over low heat, stirring occasionally, about 5 minutes or until apricots are softened. Stir in cornstarch mixture and cook, stirring constantly, until thickened, about 5 minutes. Serve warm.

❀ Makes about 2-¼ cups.

❀ 2 tablespoons contain:
Cal 40   Prot 0g   Carb 10g
Fat 0g   Chol 0mg   Sodium 1mg

2 cups apricot-mango nectar

½ cup finely chopped dried apricots

¼ cup sugar

2 tablespoons fresh lemon juice

1 tablespoon cornstarch mixed with 2 tablespoons cold water

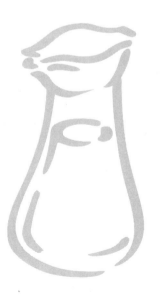

Toasted Pecan–Cinnamon Waffles with Dried Cherry Syrup

When nuts are toasted, their flavors become more pronounced and just a small amount is needed. Toasted walnuts are a great substitute.

Dried Cherry Syrup (opposite page)

2 cups all-purpose flour

1 tablespoon baking powder

¼ teaspoon salt

1 teaspoon ground cinnamon

2 cups fat-free vanilla soy milk

½ cup (4 oz.) soft silken tofu, drained and puréed

2 tablespoons vegetable oil

¼ cup chopped toasted pecans (see Note opposite)

Make syrup and keep warm. Preheat a waffle iron. Combine flour, baking powder, salt and cinnamon in a medium bowl. Stir together soy milk, tofu and oil in another bowl. Stir milk mixture into flour mixture just until combined. Stir in pecans. Spoon batter into hot waffle iron and bake according to manufacturer's directions until lightly browned.

✳ Makes about 16 (4-inch) waffles.

✳ 1 waffle and 2 tablespoons syrup contain:
Cal 143   Prot 3g   Carb 26g
Fat 4g   Chol 0mg   Sodium 134mg

Note: To toast pecans or other nuts, place nuts in a small baking pan. Place in a 350F (175C) oven for about 5 minutes, turning once, until fragrant and toasted.

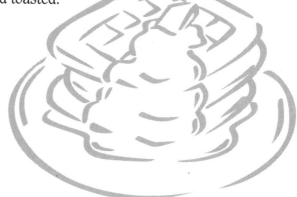

Dried Cherry Syrup

Almond extract accents the flavor of the dried cherries.

Combine apple juice, cherries, sugar and almond extract in a medium saucepan. Cook over low heat, stirring occasionally, about 5 minutes or until cherries are softened. Stir in cornstarch mixture and cook, stirring constantly, until thickened, about 5 minutes. Serve warm.

❋ Makes about 2 cups.

❋ 2 tablespoons contain:

Cal 45	Prot 0g	Carb 13g
Fat 0g	Chol 0mg	Sodium 1mg

2 cups unsweetened apple juice

¾ cup dried tart cherries, coarsely chopped

¼ cup sugar

¼ teaspoon almond extract

1 tablespoon cornstarch mixed with 2 tablespoons cold water

Banana Waffles with Banana-Maple Syrup

I prefer to eat bananas while they are still firm, but I save the ripe ones for baking. I developed this recipe when my banana supply exceeded the speed at which I was eating them. Now I let them ripen on purpose just so I have an excuse to make these waffles.

Banana-Maple Syrup (opposite page)

1-¾ cups all-purpose flour

3 tablespoons defatted soy flour

1 tablespoon baking powder

¼ teaspoon salt

½ teaspoon ground cardamom

2 cups fat-free vanilla soy milk

1 cup mashed ripe bananas (about 2 medium)

2 tablespoons vegetable oil

Make syrup and keep warm. Preheat a waffle iron. Combine flours, baking powder, salt and cardamom in a medium bowl. Stir together soy milk, bananas and oil in another bowl. Stir milk mixture into flour mixture just until combined. Spoon batter into hot waffle iron and bake according to manufacturer's directions until lightly browned.

❀ Makes about 16 (4-inch) waffles.

❀ 1 waffle and 2 tablespoons syrup contain:
Cal 156   Prot 3g   Carb 31g
Fat 3g   Chol 0mg   Sodium 131mg

Variation
Substitute cocoa-flavored soy milk for the vanilla soy milk.

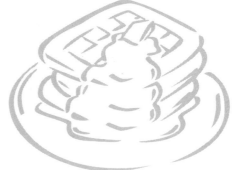

Banana-Maple Syrup

This captures the flavors of bananas Foster, with fewer calories.

Combine cornstarch and a little of the apple juice in a medium saucepan. Stir in remaining apple juice and maple syrup. Cook over low heat, stirring constantly, about 5 minutes or until thickened. Stir in banana and rum flavoring and remove from heat. Serve warm.

❋ Makes about 2 cups.

❋ 2 tablespoons contain:

Cal 70	Prot 1g	Carb 18g
Fat 0g	Chol 0mg	Sodium 2mg

1-½ tablespoons
  cornstarch

1 cup apple juice

1 cup pure
  maple syrup

1 banana, chopped

1 teaspoon
  rum flavoring

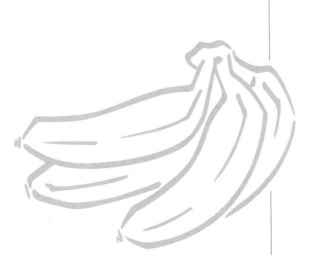

Cherry-Almond Coffeecake

If you like almonds, try this recipe using almond paste, almond extract, dried cherries and almonds; it's one of my favorites.

1 package active dry yeast

2 teaspoons sugar

¼ cup warm water (110F, 45C)

½ cup soft margarine

½ cup vanilla soy milk

2 teaspoons pure vanilla extract

½ cup packed light brown sugar

½ teaspoon salt

2 cups all-purpose flour

¾ cup whole-wheat flour

2 tablespoons defatted soy flour

¼ cup oat bran

Cherry-Almond Filling (see below)

½ cup sliced or slivered almonds

CHERRY-ALMOND FILLING

1 (7-ounce) package almond paste, cut into pieces

¾ cup (6 oz.) soft silken tofu, drained

½ cup packed light brown sugar

½ teaspoon pure almond extract

2 tablespoons all-purpose flour

1 cup dried tart cherries, chopped

Sprinkle yeast and sugar over water in a large bowl. Let stand about 5 minutes or until frothy. Beat in margarine, soy milk, vanilla, brown sugar and salt. Beat in flours and oat bran to make a soft dough. Knead on a lightly floured board until smooth and satiny. Cover and let rest while making filling.

Make filling. Grease a 13 x 9-inch nonstick baking pan. Roll out dough to a ½-inch-thick rectangle. Place dough in pan and press dough ½ inch up sides of pan.

Spread filling over dough. Sprinkle with almonds. Cover with plastic wrap and place in the refrigerator at least 2 hours or overnight.

Preheat oven to 350F (175C). Bake coffeecake about 30 minutes or until filling is softly set and edges of coffeecake are golden brown. Cool in pan on a wire rack 10 minutes. Cut into squares. Serve warm or at room temperature.

❉ Makes 12 to 15 servings.

❉ 1 serving contains:
| Cal 379 | Prot 9g | Carb 56g |
| Fat 16g | Chol 0mg | Sodium 171mg |

Cherry-Almond Filling

Combine all filling ingredients except cherries in a food processor. Process until smooth. Stir in cherries.

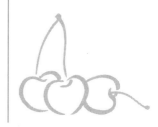

Blueberry Coffeecake

For an attractive presentation, dust the top lightly with powdered sugar just before serving.

¾ cup (6 oz.) soft silken tofu, drained

¾ cup sugar

¼ cup soft margarine

¼ cup fat-free vanilla soy milk

2 teaspoons pure vanilla extract

1-½ cups all-purpose flour

½ cup rolled oats

2 teaspoons baking powder

¼ teaspoon salt

¼ teaspoon freshly grated nutmeg

1-½ cups fresh or frozen blueberries

Preheat oven to 350F (175C). Spray a nonstick Bundt pan with nonstick cooking spray. Beat tofu in a medium bowl until smooth. Add sugar and margarine and beat until combined. Beat in soy milk and vanilla.

Combine flour, oats, baking powder, salt and nutmeg in a medium bowl. Add flour mixture to tofu mixture and beat until combined. Stir in blueberries.

Spoon mixture into prepared pan. Bake about 35 minutes or until top springs back when lightly pressed. Cool in pan 10 minutes. Serve warm.

❀ Makes 8 servings.

❀ 1 serving contains:

| Cal 256 | Prot 5g | Carb 45g |
| Fat 7g | Chol 0mg | Sodium 254mg |

Baked Breakfast Grits

If Soyrizo™ is not sold in your area, use the brand of soy sausage that is available. Serve the casserole for brunch with a fresh fruit salad.

Preheat oven to 400F (205C). Spray a 2-quart casserole dish with nonstick cooking spray. Bring grits, salt and water to a boil in a medium saucepan. Cook, stirring, until thickened, about 5 minutes. Remove from heat.

Cook soy sausage according to package directions. Stir soy sausage, chives and thyme into grits.

Beat egg whites in a medium bowl until stiff but not dry. Fold beaten egg whites into grits mixture and transfer to prepared casserole dish. Bake about 35 minutes or until puffed and browned. Serve immediately.

❈ Makes 6 servings.

❈ 1 serving contains:
| Cal 212 | Prot 10g | Carb 26g |
| Fat 7g | Chol 0mg | Sodium 464mg |

1 cup corn grits

¼ teaspoon salt

4 cups water

½ (12-oz.) package Soyrizo™ meatless soy chorizo

¼ cup minced chives

1 teaspoon dried thyme

3 egg whites

Southwestern Egg Scramble

This colorful dish will wake up hungry appetites. Combining eggs and tofu is a great way to reduce the cholesterol in an egg dish.

4 eggs

1 (12-oz.) package soft silken tofu, drained

¼ teaspoon salt

Freshly ground pepper

1 jalapeño chile, finely chopped

1 medium tomato, chopped

¼ cup chopped fresh cilantro or parsley

Beat eggs, tofu, salt and pepper together in a medium bowl; set aside. Spray a nonstick skillet with nonstick cooking spray. Add chile and tomato and cook over medium heat until softened, about 2 minutes.

Add cilantro and egg mixture. Cook, stirring gently, until egg mixture is set, about 4 minutes.

❋ Makes 4 servings.

❋ 1 serving contains:
Cal 104	Prot 11g	Carb 3g
Fat 5g	Chol 187mg	Sodium 247mg

Egg, Chile & Ham Puff

Be careful not to overbake this casserole, which has a delicate texture similar to a baked custard.

Preheat oven to 350F (175C). Spray a shallow 2-quart casserole dish with nonstick cooking spray. Heat oil in a skillet over medium heat. Add onion and cook, stirring occasionally, until softened, about 5 minutes. Add mushrooms and cook until mushrooms are softened and liquid evaporates.

Beat tofu until smooth. Beat in eggs, flour, thyme and pepper in a medium bowl. Stir in chiles, onion mixture and ham. Transfer mixture to prepared casserole dish. Bake about 20 minutes or until puffed and set.

✿ Makes 6 servings.

✿ 1 serving contains:

Cal 131	Prot 12g	Carb 9g
Fat 5g	Chol 102mg	Sodium 355mg

2 teaspoons olive oil

1 cup chopped onion

8 oz. mushrooms, sliced

1 (12.3-oz.) extra-firm low-fat silken tofu, drained

3 eggs

2 tablespoons all-purpose flour

1 teaspoon dried thyme

Freshly ground black pepper

1 (4-oz.) can chopped green chiles, drained

4 oz. cooked extra-lean ham, cut into thin strips

Breakfast Wraps

Serve these with either your own or a purchased salsa. For brunch, include an avocado-citrus salad to complete the menu.

4 oz. Soyrizo™ meatless soy chorizo or other soy sausage

4 eggs

1 tablespoon plain, unsweetened soy milk or water

2 green onions, including tops, finely chopped

2 tablespoons finely chopped red bell pepper

¼ teaspoon salt

Freshly ground black pepper

1 tablespoon margarine

4 (about 7-inch) flour tortillas, warmed (see Note, page 65)

1 medium tomato, chopped

½ cup (2 oz.) shredded Monterey jack cheese (optional)

Cook soy sausage according to package directions; set aside.

Beat together eggs, soy milk, green onions, bell pepper, salt and black pepper in a medium bowl. Melt margarine in a medium skillet over medium heat. Add egg mixture and cook, stirring gently, until eggs are set.

Spoon sausage and eggs in center of each tortilla. Top with tomato and cheese, if using. Fold one side of tortilla over filling, then fold in remaining sides. Serve warm.

❋ Makes 4 servings.

❋ 1 serving contains:

Cal 266	Prot 15g	Carb 20g
Fat 14g	Chol 200mg	Sodium 597mg

Better Pork Sausages

Because there is so little fat in these sausages, they can quickly become too browned if the heat is too high or they are cooked too long, so watch carefully.

Combine TSP and boiling water in a medium bowl. Let stand 10 minutes or until water is absorbed, stirring occasionally.

Using an electric mixer, beat in remaining ingredients until evenly combined. Using 1/3 cup for each patty, shape mixture into patties.

Spray a nonstick skillet and place over medium-low heat. Add sausages and cook, turning, about 10 minutes or until cooked through and golden brown.

❀ Makes about 12 sausages.

❀ 1 sausage contains:
Cal 77	Prot 9g	Carb 2g
Fat 4g	Chol 18mg	Sodium 192mg

7/8 cup TSP (textured soy protein)

1 cup boiling water

8 oz. lean ground pork

1 teaspoon dried thyme

1 teaspoon dried sage

½ teaspoon salt

¼ teaspoon ground cayenne

Freshly ground black pepper

Ham Strata

Feature this dish at your next brunch. Assemble it the night before and bake just before serving, if desired.

4 whole-wheat bread slices, crusts removed and slices cut into 1-inch squares

1 cup diced cooked extra-lean ham

1 cup (8 oz.) soft silken tofu, drained

3 eggs

1 cup plain, unsweetened soy milk

1 teaspoon dry mustard

2 tablespoons minced green onion

Preheat oven to 350F (175C). Spray an 8-inch-square baking pan with nonstick cooking spray. Arrange bread cubes in prepared pan. Sprinkle ham over bread.

Beat tofu until smooth. Add eggs and beat until combined. Beat in soy milk, mustard and onion. Pour over ham and bread.

Bake about 40 minutes or until set. Serve warm.

✤ Makes 6 servings.

✤ 1 serving contains:
  Cal 135   Prot 12g   Carb 12g
  Fat 5g   Chol 104mg   Sodium 520mg

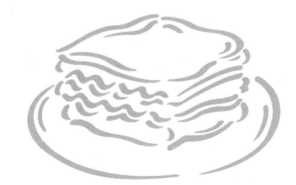

Soy Bacon Quiche

Reduce the amount of cholesterol by half but keep the protein—normally a quiche for six would have at least six eggs. Here three eggs serve six.

Preheat oven to 375F (190C). Line a 9-inch pie pan with pastry; set aside.

Spray a nonstick skillet with nonstick cooking spray. Add green onions and bell pepper and cook, stirring occasionally, over medium-low heat until softened, about 3 minutes.

Beat tofu in a medium bowl until smooth. Beat in eggs, flour, salt, pepper, bacon and cooked vegetables. Pour mixture into pastry-lined pan.

Bake about 25 minutes or until set. Let stand 5 minutes before cutting into wedges.

❋ Makes 6 servings.

❋ 1 serving contains:
| Cal 180 | Prot 5g | Carb 14g |
| Fat 11g | Chol 93mg | Sodium 365mg |

Note: Soy bacon has about half the fat as pork bacon, but it is still not a low-fat food. However, the flavor is very similar to "real" bacon. The brand—Stripples®—that I used contains egg whites.

Single crust pastry (page 129)

¼ cup chopped green onions

¼ cup finely chopped bell pepper

¾ cup (6 oz.) silken tofu, drained

3 eggs

1 tablespoon all-purpose flour

¼ teaspoon salt

Freshly ground pepper

6 slices soy bacon, cooked and crumbled (see Note, opposite)

Zucchini Frittata with Tomato-Basil Salsa

Frittata is a firm Italian omelet. Serve with the Tomato-Basil Salsa or buy a fresh salsa at your supermarket. This is an ideal dish for lunch or a light supper.

Tomato-Basil Salsa (see below)

1 cup shredded zucchini

1 cup (8 oz.) soft silken tofu, drained

3 eggs

½ teaspoon salt or to taste

2 teaspoons olive oil

¼ cup finely chopped
  red bell pepper

2 tablespoons finely chopped
  green onion

TOMATO-BASIL SALSA

2 medium tomatoes, finely chopped

2 tablespoons finely chopped fresh
  basil

1 green onion, finely chopped

1 tablespoon balsamic vinegar

1 tablespoon fresh lime juice

1 teaspoon honey

¼ teaspoon salt or to taste

Prepare salsa and set aside. Preheat broiler. Place zucchini in a paper towel and press out excess moisture. Beat tofu until smooth. Add eggs and beat well. Stir in zucchini and salt and set aside.

Heat oil in a nonstick 10-inch skillet that can go under the broiler. Add bell pepper and onion and cook over medium heat, stirring occasionally, until onion is softened, about 3 minutes.

Add egg mixture and cook until lightly browned on bottom, about 4 minutes. Place skillet under broiler, about 4 inches from heat. Broil about 3 minutes or until top is lightly browned and mixture is set. Cut into wedges to serve with salsa.

✳ Makes 6 servings.

✳ 1 serving with salsa contains:
| Cal 85 | Prot 6g | Carb 7g |
| Fat 4g | Chol 94mg | Sodium 325mg |

Tomato-Basil Salsa

Combine all ingredients in a small bowl. Makes about 1 cup.

Papaya-Strawberry Smoothie

A great breakfast on the go! This is a smooth creamy drink, almost like a milkshake. For an even thicker smoothie, use frozen strawberries.

1 cup papaya pieces

1 cup strawberries

1 (12-oz.) package soft silken tofu, drained

1 (11.5-oz.) can papaya nectar, chilled

Add all ingredients to a blender and blend until smooth. Pour into glasses and serve.

❋ Makes 4-½ cups.

❋ ½ cup contains:
| Cal 45 | Prot 3g | Carb 8g |
| Fat 0.5g | Chol 0mg | Sodium 27mg |

Variation
Almost any combination of fruit and fruit juices can be used.

Mango-Banana Smoothie

The protein powder has a slight grainy texture that is masked by the smoothness of the banana.

½ ripe mango, chopped

1 small banana, chopped

2 tablespoons vanilla soy protein powder

½ cup fat-free plain yogurt

1 cup orange juice

Add all ingredients to a blender and blend until smooth. Pour into glasses and serve.

❋ Makes 4 cups.

❋ 1 cup contains:
| Cal 97 | Prot 4g | Carb 21g |
| Fat 0.8g | Chol 2mg | Sodium 23mg |

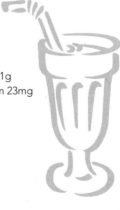

desserts

ESSERTS ARE THE PERFECT PLACE TO START adding soy products to your cooking! Many of the desserts in this section, such as Creamy Cherry Parfait and Easy Mocha Mousse, require no cooking at all. Both tofu and soy cream cheese are used in these recipes. If you like, use low-fat dairy cream cheese instead of the soy cream cheese the first time you make these desserts.

Feel free to create your own dessert by varying the flavors or embellishments to reflect your taste.

You'll feel better about offering these desserts more often. The baked goods contain tofu, defatted soy flour, soy milk or a combination of these ingredients. You will find that items baked with soy need fewer eggs and contain less fat but are still moist. Only a few of the recipes contain eggs—especially helpful for those who are concerned about their cholesterol intake. Most of the baked goods are actually moister the second day.

Don't tell family and friends that you are cooking with soy until *after* they have told you how delicious your desserts are. Then watch their surprise!

Rhubarb-Strawberry Custard Pie

A favorite combination at our house is rhubarb and strawberries. The creamy topping blends well with the fruit flavors of the filling.

1-½ cups sliced rhubarb

1-½ cups sliced strawberries

½ cup sugar

1-½ tablespoons cornstarch

1 unbaked (9-inch) Crust (opposite page)

CUSTARD TOPPING:

1 (12-oz.) package firm low-fat silken tofu

½ cup fat-free vanilla soy milk

3 tablespoons all-purpose flour

4 tablespoons sugar

2 tablespoons fresh lemon juice

1 tablespoon grated lemon zest

½ teaspoon freshly grated nutmeg

Preheat oven to 400F (205C). Make filling: Combine rhubarb, strawberries, sugar and cornstarch in a medium bowl. Transfer rhubarb mixture to pie shell. Bake 20 minutes.

Meanwhile, make topping: Process tofu, soy milk, flour, 3 tablespoons of the sugar, the lemon juice, lemon zest and nutmeg in a food processor until smooth. Pour tofu mixture over hot filling. Sprinkle with remaining 1 tablespoon sugar.

Reduce oven temperature to 350F (175C). Bake about 20 minutes or until topping is browned. Cool on a wire rack before cutting. Refrigerate leftovers.

✺ Makes 6 to 8 servings.

✺ 1 serving contains:
Cal 176	Prot 5g	Carb 36g
Fat 2g	Chol 0mg	Sodium 23mg

Better Pecan Pie

Tofu and condensed milk team up to make a creamy filling, almost like a custard—without the eggs.

Prepare crust. Preheat oven to 350F (175C).

Process tofu and maple syrup in a food processor until combined. Add condensed milk, flour and vanilla and process until smooth. Stir in pecans.

Pour filling into crust. Bake about 40 minutes or until filling is set. Refrigerate until chilled before cutting. Refrigerate leftovers.

❋ Makes 8 servings.

❋ 1 serving contains:
| Cal 479 | Prot 9g | Carb 49g |
| Fat 4g | Chol 6mg | Sodium 218mg |

Crust
Combine flour and salt in a food processor. Add half of the butter or margarine and process until mixture resembles coarse crumbs. Add remaining butter or margarine and process until butter is the size of small peas. Stir in enough water that mixture holds together and can be formed into a ball. Cover with plastic wrap and refrigerate 30 minutes.

Roll out dough on a lightly floured board to an 11-inch circle. Fit circle into a 9-inch pie pan. Fold edges under and flute.

Crust (see below)

1 (12.3-oz.) extra-firm low-fat silken tofu, drained

½ cup pure maple syrup

½ cup nonfat condensed milk

3 tablespoons all-purpose flour

1 tablespoon pure vanilla extract

1-½ cups pecan halves

CRUST:

1-½ cups all-purpose flour

¼ teaspoon salt

½ cup butter or margarine, chilled

About 4 tablespoons water

Berry Cobbler

Frozen berries are almost always less expensive than fresh ones and they enable you to make this dessert in any season. However, if you put the crust over frozen berries, the filling will still be undercooked when the crust is baked. Cooking the berry filling in the microwave first saves time, because the berries don't have to be thawed.

The pastry is delicate and is easier to handle after a few minutes of chilling.

Yogurt Pastry (see below)

2 cups frozen boysenberries

2 cups frozen blueberries

½ cup fructose or ¾ cup sugar

2 tablespoons cornstarch

YOGURT PASTRY:

1 cup all-purpose flour

¼ teaspoon baking powder

1/8 teaspoon baking soda

¼ cup soft margarine

½ cup soy yogurt

1 teaspoon pure vanilla extract

Preheat oven to 375F (190C). Prepare pastry, wrap in plastic wrap and chill in the freezer while preparing filling.

Combine berries in an 8-inch-square, microwave-safe baking dish. Combine fructose and cornstarch in a small bowl. Sprinkle fructose mixture over frozen berries and toss to combine. Microwave berries on HIGH 3 minutes and stir. Microwave about 2 minutes more or until bubbly and stir again.

Roll out pastry on a lightly floured surface to a 9-inch square and fit over filling. Cut slits to allow steam to escape. Bake about 30 minutes until crust is lightly browned and filling is bubbly.

Yogurt Pastry
Combine flour, baking powder and baking soda in a food processor. Add margarine and process until crumbly. Add soy yogurt and vanilla and process until combined. Shape into a ball. Chill dough for approximately 30 minutes to make it easier to handle.

❋ Makes 5 or 6 servings.

❋ 1 serving contains:
Cal 269   Prot 3g   Carb 49g
Fat 8g   Chol 0mg   Sodium 113mg

Creamy Cherry Parfait

So quick, easy and delicious, this is pretty enough for a special meal, but don't wait—serve it any time!!

Combine crumbs and pecans, if using; set aside.

Process tofu and cream cheese in a food processor until smooth. Add honey, kirschwasser, if using, and almond extract and process until combined.

Sprinkle 1 tablespoon of crumbs in the bottom of each of 6 parfait glasses. Add a layer of tofu mixture, then a layer of the pie filling. Repeat layers, ending with pie filling. Cover and refrigerate until chilled or up to 24 hours.

❀ Makes 6 servings.

❀ 1 serving contains:
Cal 297   Prot 9g   Carb 46g
Fat 10g   Chol 0mg   Sodium 157mg

Variation
Cherry Cheesecake: Sprinkle 1 package unflavored gelatin over ½ cup orange juice in a small saucepan. Let stand until softened, about 5 minutes. Stir over low heat until dissolved. Stir gelatin mixture into tofu mixture. Add 2 tablespoons softened butter or margarine to crumbs and press into the bottom of an 8-inch springform pan. Pour tofu mixture over crumbs. Spoon pie filling over the top. Cover and refrigerate until firm, about 3 hours.

¾ cup graham-cracker crumbs

2 tablespoons ground toasted pecans (optional) (see Note, page 110)

1 (12.3-oz.) package extra-firm low-fat silken tofu, drained

1 (8-oz.) package plain soy cream cheese or 8 oz. whipped low-fat cream cheese

¼ cup honey

1 tablespoon kirschwasser (optional)

½ teaspoon pure almond extract

1 (20-oz.) can light cherry pie filling

Maple Rice Pudding

So easy to do—no baking is required. I always cook extra rice and keep it in the freezer for quick casseroles and desserts such as this one. Rice can be thawed quickly in the microwave.

1 (12.3-oz.) package extra-firm low-fat silken tofu, drained

¼ cup pure maple syrup

1-½ teaspoons pure vanilla extract

1 teaspoon ground cinnamon

¼ teaspoon ground allspice

1 cup dried cranberries

1-¼ cups cooked long-grain white rice

¼ teaspoon freshly grated nutmeg

¼ cup sliced almonds, toasted (see Note, page 110)

Process tofu in a food processor until smooth; add syrup, vanilla, cinnamon and allspice and process until combined. Add cranberries and pulse to chop. Stir in rice.

Transfer mixture to a serving dish. Sprinkle with nutmeg and almonds. Cover and refrigerate until chilled.

❀ Makes 4 servings.

❀ 1 serving contains:
Cal 242   Prot 9g   Carb 39g
Fat 6g   Chol 0mg   Sodium 157mg

Variation
Omit dried cranberries. Serve with sliced fresh strawberries.

Easy Mocha Mousse

Mocha is a blend of coffee and chocolate; together the flavors contribute to a delectable and easy dessert. Add the optional garnishes for a beautiful presentation.

Melt chocolate chips with maple syrup in a double boiler over simmering water, stirring occasionally. Combine tofu and cream cheese in a food processor and process until smooth. Add chocolate mixture, coffee and vanilla and pulse until mixed.

Spoon into 6 dessert dishes. Cover and refrigerate until chilled or up to 24 hours. Garnish with whipped cream and chocolate-covered coffee beans, if desired.

❋ Makes 6 servings.

❋ 1 serving contains:
| Cal 419 | Prot 10g | Carb 48g |
| Fat 24g | Chol 21mg | Sodium 157mg |

1 (12-oz.) package semisweet chocolate chips

¼ cup pure maple syrup

1 (12.3-oz.) package extra-firm low-fat silken tofu, drained

1 (8-oz.) package soy cream cheese or 8 oz. whipped low-fat cream cheese

1 tablespoon instant espresso powder dissolved in 2 tablespoons hot water

1 tablespoon pure vanilla extract

Whipping cream, whipped, and chocolate-covered coffee beans for garnish (optional)

Spicy Pumpkin Mousse

Serve instead of the traditional pumpkin pie. No one will guess that the secret ingredient is tofu.

1 cup orange juice

¾ cup sugar

1 (¼-oz.) envelope unflavored gelatin

1 (15-oz.) can pumpkin

1 teaspoon ground cinnamon

½ teaspoon ground cloves

½ teaspoon ground allspice

¼ teaspoon freshly grated nutmeg

1 (12.3-oz.) package extra-firm low-fat silken tofu, drained

2 tablespoons finely chopped pecans, toasted (see Note, page 110)

Add orange juice and sugar to a small saucepan. Sprinkle gelatin over juice. Let stand until softened, about 1 minute. Stir over low heat until gelatin is completely dissolved.

Process pumpkin, spices and tofu in a food processor or blender until combined. Add gelatin mixture and process until combined.

Pour pumpkin mixture into 6 dessert dishes. Sprinkle with pecans. Cover and refrigerate 3 hours or until firm.

❋ Makes 6 servings.

❋ 1 serving contains:
Cal 183	Prot 6g	Carb 37g
Fat 3g	Chol 0mg	Sodium 157mg

Variation

Pumpkin Cheesecake: Coat an 8-inch-square pan or a 9-inch springform pan with 2 teaspoons soft margarine. Sprinkle with about ½ cup graham cracker crumbs and turn pan to coat. Pour pumpkin mixture into prepared pan. Top with pecans. Refrigerate until set. Cut into pieces to serve.

Strawberry Trifle

We credit the English for creating trifle, which was originated to use cake left over from the previous day's tea. If fresh berries aren't in season, substitute frozen ones.

Process tofu and cream cheese in a food processor until smooth. Add orange juice, Grand Marnier, sugar, vanilla and orange zest and process until combined.

Sprinkle half of the cake in the bottom of a 1-quart glass serving dish. Top with half of the strawberries. Repeat layers, ending with strawberries. Top with whipped cream, if desired. Cover and refrigerate until chilled or up to 8 hours.

❊ Makes 6 to 8 servings.

❊ 1 serving contains:
| Cal 304 | Prot 11g | Carb 46g |
| Fat 8g | Chol 21mg | Sodium 45mg |

1 (12-oz.) package soft silken tofu, drained

8 oz. soft low-fat cream cheese

¼ cup orange juice

2 tablespoons Grand Marnier

¼ cup sugar

1 teaspoon pure vanilla extract

1 tablespoon grated orange zest

3 cups angel food cake or pound-cake cubes

1 pint strawberries, washed, hulled and sliced

Whipped cream (optional)

Crepes with Creamy Peach Filling and Toasted Almonds

Let the batter stand at least one hour before cooking the crepes. Crepes can be cooked the day before, covered and stored in the refrigerator. To make separating them easier, place a piece of waxed paper between each crepe.

CREPES:

½ cup all-purpose flour

1 tablespoon sugar (optional)

¾ cup fat-free vanilla soy milk

2 egg whites

2 tablespoons soft margarine, melted, or vegetable oil

1 teaspoon pure vanilla extract

Pinch of salt

CREAMY FILLING:

1 (12.3-oz.) package extra-firm low-fat silken tofu, drained

1 (8-oz.) package plain soy cream cheese or 8 oz. whipped low-fat cream cheese

¼ cup sugar

½ teaspoon pure vanilla extract

½ teaspoon pure almond extract

¼ cup fat-free vanilla soy milk

TO ASSEMBLE:

4 fresh peaches or 3 cups frozen sliced peaches, thawed

1 tablespoon freshly squeezed lemon juice

2 tablespoons granulated sugar

2 tablespoons powdered sugar

¼ cup sliced almonds

Make crepe batter: Combine all ingredients in a blender or food processor and process until smooth. Pour batter into a large glass measuring cup or pitcher. Cover and refrigerate 1 hour.

Make filling: Process tofu and cream cheese in a food processor until smooth. Add sugar, vanilla and almond extract and process until combined. Add soy milk and process until combined. Transfer to a bowl, cover and refrigerate until chilled.

Heat a well-seasoned or nonstick 7-inch crepe pan or skillet over medium. Spray with nonstick cooking spray. Stir batter. Pour about 3 tablespoons of batter into center of pan, tilting pan quickly so batter covers bottom completely. Cook until bottom of crepe is brown. Turn crepe and cook until bottom of crepe is light brown. Remove crepe to a plate and continue making crepes with remaining batter. Put a sheet of waxed paper between each crepe. Makes 12 crepes.

To assemble: Preheat oven to 425F (220C). Spray a baking sheet with nonstick cooking spray. Peel peaches and cut into thin wedges. Toss with lemon juice and granulated sugar. Stir peaches into filling. Place a crepe on a work surface, spoon 1/6 filling on one half of crepe; fold in half, then quarters, enclosing filling. Place filled crepe on baking sheet. Repeat with remaining crepes and filling. Sift powdered sugar over crepes and sprinkle with almonds. Bake 20 minutes, until filling is hot and almonds are toasted.

❋ Makes 6 servings.

❋ 1 serving contains:
Cal 163	Prot 6g	Carb 18g
Fat 8g	Chol 11mg	Sodium 147mg

Rhubarb Cheese Pie

A wonderful springtime dessert when rhubarb is in season, it can be made any time if you use frozen rhubarb. The filling will remind you of cheesecake.

Crust (page 129), unbaked, in a 9-inch tart pan

1 cup (8 oz.) extra-firm low-fat silken tofu, drained

½ cup (4 oz.) low-fat cream cheese

1 egg

2 teaspoons pure vanilla extract

2 cups chopped rhubarb

⅓ cup sugar or to taste

2 tablespoons water

Preheat oven to 375F (190C). Line crust with foil and fill with pie weights or dried beans. Bake 10 minutes. Remove foil and weights and set aside. Place crust on a wire rack to cool while making topping.

Process tofu and cream cheese in a food processor until smooth. Add egg, vanilla and 1 tablespoon of the sugar; process until combined. Pour tofu mixture into partially baked crust. Bake 10 minutes or until filling is set.

Combine rhubarb, remaining sugar and water in a medium saucepan over medium heat. Cook, stirring, until rhubarb is soft and falls apart. Cool slightly and spoon over filling. Refrigerate until chilled. Cut into wedges to serve.

❀ Makes 6 to 8 servings.

❀ 1 serving contains:
Cal 133   Prot 6g   Carb 16g
Fat 5g   Chol 42mg   Sodium 105mg

Variation
Top tart with fresh sliced strawberries and brush with melted currant jelly instead of making the rhubarb topping.

Brownies

Make chocolate lovers even happier and top these with the creamy Chocolate Frosting (page 150). The silken tofu replaces much of the margarine found in regular brownie recipes.

Preheat oven to 350F (175C). Spray a nonstick 8-inch-square pan with nonstick cooking spray.

Beat tofu in a medium bowl until smooth. Add sugar, margarine and vanilla and beat until combined.

Combine flour, cocoa, baking powder and salt in a small bowl. Add flour mixture to tofu mixture and beat until combined. Pour mixture into prepared pan.

Bake 25 to 30 minutes or until top springs back when lightly pressed. Cool in pan 10 minutes. Remove from pan and cut into squares.

❀ Makes 16 (2-inch) squares.

❀ 1 square contains:

Cal 93	Prot 2g	Carb 15g
Fat 3g	Chol 0mg	Sodium 78mg

½ cup (4 oz.) silken tofu, drained

¾ cup sugar

¼ cup soft margarine

2 teaspoons pure vanilla extract

¾ cup all-purpose flour

½ cup unsweetened cocoa powder

½ teaspoon baking powder

¼ teaspoon salt

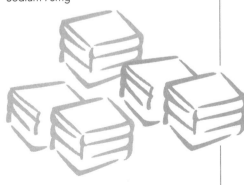

Carrot Spice Cake

A dense, moist cake packed with carrots, pineapple and pecans that is destined to become a favorite.

½ cup crushed pineapple, drained and juice reserved

¾ cup (6 oz.) soft silken tofu, drained and puréed

¾ cup sugar

¼ cup vegetable oil

1 teaspoon pure vanilla extract

2-½ cups all-purpose flour

¼ cup defatted soy flour

2 teaspoons baking powder

½ teaspoon baking soda

½ teaspoon salt

1-½ teaspoons ground allspice

1 teaspoon ground cinnamon

1 cup grated carrots

½ cup chopped pecans

Creamy Vanilla Frosting (page 151)

Preheat oven to 350F (175C). Spray 2 (9-inch) round baking pans with nonstick cooking spray.

Add water to reserved pineapple juice to make ¾ cup. Beat tofu, sugar, oil and vanilla in a medium bowl until smooth. Stir in pineapple juice. Combine flours, baking powder, baking soda, salt, allspice and cinnamon; beat into tofu mixture until combined. Stir in carrots, pineapple and pecans. Pour into prepared pans and smooth tops.

Bake about 30 minutes or until tops spring back when pressed. Cool in pans on a wire rack 10 minutes. Remove from pans and place on a wire rack to finish cooling.

Place 1 layer topside down on a serving plate. Spread with frosting and top with remaining layer topside up. Frost top of cake with remaining frosting. Refrigerate until chilled. Cut into wedges to serve. Refrigerate leftovers.

❀ Makes 12 servings.

❀ 1 serving contains:
Cal 364   Prot 7g   Carb 51g
Fat 6g   Chol 0mg   Sodium 141mg

Quick Lemon Poppy-Seed Cake

The cake is quite moist and needs no frosting. Dust with powdered sugar, if desired. For a special occasion, spread a purchased lemon curd between layers.

Preheat oven to 350F (175C). Spray 2 (9-inch) round baking pans with nonstick cooking spray.

Blend together cake mix, tofu, water, lemon juice, lemon zest and poppy seeds. Beat 2 minutes.

Pour batter into prepared pans and bake 30 to 35 minutes or until centers spring back when lightly pressed. Cool in pans on a wire rack 10 minutes. Remove from pans and place on a wire rack to finish cooling. Cut into wedges to serve.

❀ Makes 12 servings.

❀ 1 serving contains:
Cal 200	Prot 3g	Carb 35g
Fat 6g	Chol 0mg	Sodium 300mg

1 (18.25-oz.) package lemon cake mix

1 cup soft silken tofu, puréed

½ cup water

2 tablespoons fresh lemon juice

1 tablespoon grated lemon zest

2 tablespoons poppy seeds

Variations
1. Use a white cake mix instead of lemon.
2. Use a Bundt pan. Bake 35 to 40 minutes or until cake springs back when pressed lightly.

Gingerbread

This rich, moist gingerbread is even better the second day. Try topping top it with sliced strawberries or peaches, lemon sauce or vanilla ice cream.

1 cup (8 oz.) soft silken tofu, puréed

½ cup molasses

¼ cup sugar

¼ cup soft margarine

1 cup all-purpose flour

½ cup whole-wheat flour

1 teaspoon baking powder

½ teaspoon baking soda

¼ teaspoon salt

2 teaspoons ground ginger

1 teaspoon ground cinnamon

½ teaspoon ground cloves

Preheat oven to 350F (175C). Spray a nonstick 8-inch-square pan with nonstick cooking spray.

Beat tofu, molasses, sugar and margarine in a medium bowl until smooth.

Combine flours, baking powder, baking soda, salt, ginger, cinnamon and cloves in a medium bowl. Add flour mixture to tofu mixture and beat until combined. Pour mixture into prepared pan.

Bake about 35 minutes or until top springs back when lightly pressed. Cool in pan 10 minutes. Remove from pan and cut into 16 (2-inch) squares.

❀ Makes 16 squares.

❀ 1 square contains:

Cal 112	Prot 2g	Carb 19g
Fat 3g	Chol 0mg	Sodium 141mg

Applesauce Spice Bars

Sprinkle the top with powdered sugar or ice with Butterscotch Frosting (page 150). The bars are moister on the second day.

Preheat oven to 350F (175C). Spray a nonstick 13 x 9-inch baking pan with nonstick cooking spray.

Beat tofu, sugar and margarine in a medium bowl until smooth. Beat in applesauce until combined.

Combine flour, baking powder, baking soda, salt, cinnamon and allspice in a medium bowl. Add flour mixture to tofu mixture and beat until combined. Stir in walnuts and raisins. Pour mixture into prepared pan.

Bake about 35 minutes or until top springs back when lightly pressed. Cool in pan 10 minutes. Remove from pan and cut into bars.

❀ Makes 16 (3 x 2-inch) bars.

❀ 1 bar contains:

| Cal 200 | Prot 4g | Carb 34g |
| Fat 6g | Chol 0mg | Sodium 247mg |

1-¼ cups (10 oz.) soft tofu, drained

1 cup packed light brown sugar

¼ cup soft margarine

1-½ cups applesauce

3 cups all-purpose flour

2 teaspoons baking powder

1 teaspoon baking soda

½ teaspoon salt

2 teaspoons ground cinnamon

2 teaspoons ground allspice

½ cup chopped walnuts

½ cup raisins

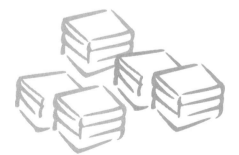

Strawberry "Ice Cream"

A truly refreshing frozen dessert. Make it doubly good by serving it with Brownies (page 139).

1-½ (12.3-oz.) packages soft silken tofu, drained

2 ripe bananas

3 cups strawberries, washed and trimmed

2 cups fat-free vanilla soy milk

¾ cup honey

Juice of 1 lime

2 tablespoons pure vanilla extract

Process all ingredients in batches in a blender until strawberries are puréed. Pour into an ice cream maker and freeze according to manufacturer's directions.

Makes about 2 quarts, 8 servings.

1 serving contains:
| Cal 182 | Prot 5g | Carb 39g |
| Fat 2g | Chol 0mg | Sodium 38mg |

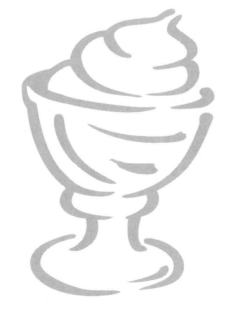

Chocolate "Ice Cream"

I like to make small batches of frozen desserts in my small hand-cranked, non-electric ice cream maker, which has a special insert that is placed in the freezer about 12 hours before it is needed. In summer, I return the empty insert to the freezer immediately —so it will be ready for the next batch.

Process all ingredients in a blender until smooth. Pour into an ice cream maker and freeze according to manufacturer's directions.

❈ Makes about 2-½ cups.

❈ ½ cup contains:
Cal 135	Prot 5g	Carb 27g
Fat 1g	Chol 0mg	Sodium 61mg

Tip: The calories and richness of the dessert will vary depending on the chocolate syrup that you choose. Fruit- or nut-flavored chocolate syrups add interesting flavors.

1 (12.3-oz.) package firm low-fat silken tofu, drained

½ cup low-fat chocolate soy milk

¼ cup honey

¼ cup chocolate syrup

2 tablespoons pure vanilla extract

Chocolate Granola Bars

The crunchy goodness of granola is combined with luscious chocolate for a great snack.

3 cups fruit-and-nut granola

½ cup soynuts

½ cup finely chopped dried apricots

1 (12-oz.) package semisweet chocolate chips

¼ cup fat-free vanilla soy milk

¼ cup honey

2 teaspoons pure vanilla extract

Line an 8-inch square pan with foil and butter foil. Combine granola, soynuts and apricots in a medium heatproof bowl; set aside.

Melt chocolate with soy milk, honey and vanilla in a small pan over low heat, stirring constantly.

Pour chocolate mixture over granola mixture and stir until coated. Press into prepared pan. Refrigerate until firm.

Cut into 2-inch squares. Store in refrigerator in an airtight container.

❋ Makes 16 (2-inch) squares.

❋ 1 square contains:
Cal 255   Prot 5g   Carb 34g
Fat 13g   Chol 0mg   Sodium 6mg

Orange Raisin Balls

A chewy confection with rich orange flavors, these can be kept in the refrigerator up to a week or frozen up to a month.

Combine raisins, crumbs, powdered sugar and orange peel in a medium bowl. Stir in orange extract and enough soy milk to hold mixture together. Refrigerate until firm enough to shape into balls, about 30 minutes.

Place coconut in a shallow bowl. Shape by tablespoonfuls into balls. Roll balls in coconut, pressing in coconut.

Store in refrigerator.

❋ Makes about 30 balls.

❋ 1 ball contains:
| Cal 48 | Prot 0g | Carb 9g |
| Fat 1g | Chol 0mg | Sodium 21mg |

1 cup golden raisins, chopped

½ cup graham-cracker crumbs

½ cup powdered sugar

1 tablespoon grated orange peel

¼ teaspoon orange extract

About ¼ cup fat-free vanilla soy milk

1 cup shredded coconut

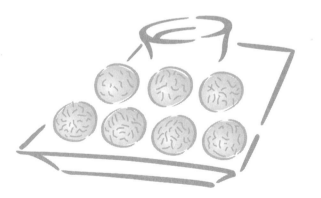

Cranberry-Cereal Bars

Dried cranberries add color and flavor to these crunchy bars.

5 cups crisp rice cereal

1 cup dried cranberries

¾ cup honey

½ cup sugar

1-½ cups roasted soynut butter

2 teaspoons pure vanilla extract

Line a 13 x 9-inch baking pan with foil and butter foil; set aside. Combine cereal and cranberries in a large heatproof bowl; set aside.

Combine honey and sugar in a medium saucepan. Cook over medium heat, stirring constantly, until sugar dissolves. Remove from heat.

Stir in soynut butter and vanilla until combined. Pour over cereal mixture, stirring until combined. Press into prepared pan. Refrigerate until firm. Cut into 2 x 1-inch bars.

❀ Makes 48 bars.

❀ 1 bar contains:
Cal 89	Prot 2g	Carb 15g
Fat 3g	Chol 0mg	Sodium 65mg

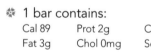

No-Bake Chocolate Cookies

These are so good and easy that you might want to double the recipe. Kids love them for snacks and these cookies are full of nutrition, not empty calories.

Line a baking sheet with waxed paper; set aside. Combine sugar and cocoa in a medium saucepan. Stir in soy milk and margarine. Bring to a full rolling boil over medium heat, stirring constantly. Stir in soynut butter, oats and vanilla. Remove from heat. Stir until well blended.

Drop warm oat mixture by spoonfuls onto waxed paper. Chill until firm. Refrigerate leftovers.

❀ Makes about 20 cookies.

❀ 1 cookie contains:

Cal 78	Prot 2g	Carb 12g
Fat 3g	Chol 0mg	Sodium 27mg

¾ cup sugar

2 tablespoons unsweetened cocoa powder

¼ cup fat-free vanilla soy milk

2 tablespoons soft margarine

¼ cup roasted soynut butter

1-¼ cups rolled oats

1 teaspoon pure vanilla extract

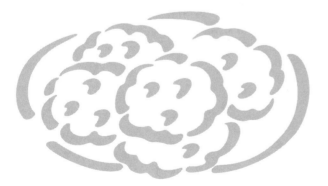

Chocolate Frosting

Creamy and full of chocolate flavor, this is good on cakes and bar cookies, or even by the spoonful!

1 cup fat-free vanilla soy milk

¼ cup all-purpose flour

½ cup sugar

1 tablespoon pure vanilla extract

6 oz. (1 cup) semisweet chocolate chips, melted and cooled

Blend a little of the soy milk and flour in a small saucepan until smooth. Stir in remaining soy milk. Cook, stirring, over medium-low heat until smooth and thick, about 5 minutes. Transfer to a bowl and refrigerate until chilled, about 30 minutes.

Beat in sugar and vanilla until sugar is dissolved, about 5 minutes. Beat in chocolate until smooth. Refrigerate until a good spreading consistency, about 30 minutes.

Makes about 2 cups.

2 tablespoons contain:
Cal 89	Prot 1g	Carb 15g
Fat 3g	Chol 0mg	Sodium 3mg

Variation

Butterscotch Frosting: Substitute butterscotch chips for chocolate chips.

Creamy Vanilla Frosting

Like many products made with soy, the flavor of this frosting is even better the next day.

Beat all ingredients in a medium bowl until smooth. Refrigerate until a good spreading consistency, about 30 minutes.

❋ Makes about 1-½ cups.

❋ 2 tablespoons contain:
Cal 93	Prot 2g	Carb 13g
Fat 3g	Chol 11mg	Sodium 68mg

1-½ cups marshmallow creme

1 (8-oz.) package plain soy cream cheese

1 tablespoon pure vanilla extract

Maple-Soynut Butter Balls

Roasted soybeans are sometimes called soynuts. *Soynut butter can be used in recipes that call for peanut butter, but because it has less fat, you will need to modify the recipes somewhat. You get two forms of soy in these nutritious and delicious confections.*

1-¼ cups vanilla-flavored soy powder

1 cup roasted soynut butter

1 cup maple syrup or honey

1-¼ cups finely chopped raisins

½ cup flaked coconut

Stir together soy powder, soynut butter, maple syrup, raisins and coconut in a medium bowl. Refrigerate until firm enough to shape into balls, about 30 minutes.

Shape by tablespoonfuls into balls. Store balls in the refrigerator in an airtight container.

❋ Makes about 45 balls.

❋ 1 ball contains:
| Cal 75 | Prot 3g | Carb 39g |
| Fat 2g | Chol 0mg | Sodium 38mg |

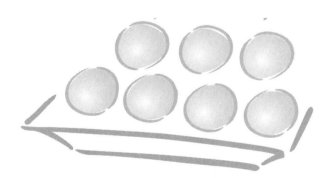

Mail-Order Sources for Soyfoods

In addition to the mail-order sources listed below, check the Internet for web sites that offer soyfoods.

Local healthfood stores and Asian markets are good sources for soyfood products in your area.

Apple Valley Mail Order
9067 U. S. 31
Berrien Springs, MI 49103
800-237-7436
Extensive list of soy products; catalog

Country Life Natural Foods
P.O. Box 489
Pullman, MI 49450
616-236-5011
Email 74532,1631@compuserve.com
Extensive list of soy products; catalog

Crusoe Island Natural Store
267 Route 89 S.
Savannah, NY 13146
800-724-2233
Organic soybeans and soy flour; catalog

Harvest Direct
P.O. Box 988
Knoxville, TN 37901-0988
423-523-2304
Extensive list of soy products; catalog

Shiloh Farms, Inc.
P.O. Box 97
White Sulphur Springs, AR 72768-0097
501-298-3297
Organic soybeans and soy flour; catalog

Other Sources

American Soybean Association
540 Maryville Centre Dr., Ste. 390
St. Louis, MO 63141
800-688-7692

Eden Foods, Inc.
701 Tecumseh Rd.
Clinton, MI 49236
517-456-7424

Soyfoods Center
P.O. Box 234
Lafayette, CA 94549-0234
Individual soy bibliographies available

United Soybean Board
P.O. Box 419200
St. Louis, MO 63141
800-989-8721

U.S. Soyfoods Directory
Indiana Soybean Development Council
4816 N. Pennsylvania St.
Indianapolis, IN 46205
http://www.soyfoods.com

INDEX

Main entries in **bold** are the major chapter headings.

A

allergies, to soyfoods, xiv
analogs (meat alternatives), xxiii
Appetizers
  artichoke-stuffed mushrooms, 4
  barbecued tofu bites, 13
  blue cheese & tofu spread, 3
  crab quesadillas, 9
  dilled salmon spread, 5
  roasted bell pepper & tofu spread, 2
  roasted eggplant spread, 7
  smoked salmon rolls, 8
  southwestern hummus, 12
  tofu dip, 1
  tuna dip, 6
  vegetable-cheese filo slices, 10–11
apples
  apple bread, 99
  apple-cabbage slaw, 45
  applesauce spice bars, 143
apricots
  apricot & currant drop scones, 104
  double-apricot syrup, 109
artichokes
  artichoke-stuffed mushrooms, 4
  tuna dip, 6
Asian cultures, health benefits from soyfoods,
  xi, xii, xiii
asparagus, mushroom bake, 85
avocado
  dressing, 48
  papaya salsa, 64
  sauce, 9

B

bacon, soy
  quiche, 123
bananas
  ginger banana bread, 100
  mango smoothie, 126
  maple syrup, 113
  waffles, 112

bell peppers
  roasting, 2
  stuffed, 56
blue cheese
  dressing, 47
  onion-cheese strudel, 66–67
blueberries
  berry cobbler, 130
  coffeecake, 116
  pancakes, 106–107
boysenberries, berry cobbler, 130
bread machine, making spiced yeast bread
  with, 102–103
Breads, 91. *See also* muffins
  apple bread, 99
  apricot & currant drop scones, 104
  cornbread, 93
  cream biscuits, 94
  dried cranberry scones, 101
  French bread crisps, 5
  ginger banana bread, 100
  spiced fruit & nut yeast bread, 102–103
Breakfast dishes, 105
  baked breakfast grits, 117
  banana waffles with banana-maple syrup,
    112
  blueberry pancakes with orange-maple
    syrup, 106–107
  cherry-almond coffeecake, 114–115
  egg, chile & ham puff, 119
  ham strata, 122
  pecan-cinnamon waffles with cherry syrup,
    110–111
  pork sausages, 121
  smoothies, 126
  southwestern egg scramble, 118
  soy bacon quiche, 123
  whole-wheat pancakes with double-apricot
    syrup, 108–109
  zucchini frittata with tomato-basil salsa,
    124–125
breast cancer, health benefits of soyfoods, xi, xii

broccoli soup, creamy, 24
bulgur
  casserole, 86
  vegetable burgers, 52–53
buttermilk
  blue cheese dressing, 47
  dressing, 43

C

cabbage-apple slaw, 45
cakes
  blueberry coffeecake, 116
  carrot spice cake, 140
  cherry-almond coffeecake, 114–115
  lemon poppy-seed cake, 141
calcium
  loss, soyfoods helping to prevent, xii–xiii
  soyfoods as good source of, xix–xx
cancer prevention, xi–xii
  anticancer chemicals in soyfoods, xii
  Asian countries' low cancer rates, xi–xii
canned soybeans, using, xxiii
cannellini beans
  vegetarian chili, 30
  white bean & tofu salad, 32
carrot spice cake, 140
caseinate (milk protein), xxiv, 9
cheeses, soy, xxiv
  chiles rellenos, 73
  crab quesadillas, 9
  corn muffins, 92
  jalapeño-flavored cheese sauce, 89
  mocha mousse, 133
  twice-baked potatoes, 88
cherries
  cheesecake, 131
  cherry-almond coffeecake, 114–115
  creamy parfait, 131
  dried cherry syrup, 111
chicken
  baked tofu & noodle salad, 38
  green chile stew, 17
  roasted vegetable pasta, 55
  tempeh curry, 50
children, recommended intake of soyfoods, xiv
chiles
  avocado sauce, 9
  chicken–green chile stew, 17
  corn muffins, 92
  egg, green chiles & ham puff, 119

rellenos, 73
roasting, 2
shrimp miso soup, 18
southwestern egg scramble, 118
southwestern hummus, 12
two-bean & corn salad, 37
chili
  black bean, 28–29
  vegetarian, 30
chocolate
  brownies, 138
  frosting, 150
  granola bars, 146
  "ice cream," 145
  mocha mousse, 133
  no-bake cookies, 149
cholesterol, soyfoods that lower, x–xi, xv
chorizo, soy
  baked breakfast grits, 117
  breakfast wraps, 120
clot formation, soyfoods reduce, xi
colon cancer, soyfoods reduce risk of, xi, xii
cookware, nonstick, 90
corn
  green soybeans, tomatoes and, 90
  muffins, 92
  two-bean salad, 37
couscous, pilaf with green soybeans, 87
crabmeat
  crab bisque, 26–27
  crab Louie, 35
  quesadilla with avocado sauce, 9
cranberries
  cereal bars, 148
  cranberry-pumpkin muffins, 98
  dried cranberry scones, 101
  maple rice pudding, 132
cream cheese, soy, xxiv
  cherry cheesecake, 94
  cream biscuits, 84
  creamy cherry parfait, 131
  smoked salmon rolls, 8
  strawberry trifle, 135
  vanilla frosting, 151
crepes
  creamy peach filling for, 136
  salmon, 60–61
currants
  apricot & currant drop scones, 104
  pecan muffins, 95

D

Desserts, 127
  applesauce spice bars, 143
  berry cobbler, 130
  carrot spicecake, 140
  cherry cheesecake, 131
  chocolate brownies, 139
  chocolate chip cookies, no-bake, 149
  chocolate frosting, 150
  chocolate granola bars, 146
  chocolate "ice cream," 145
  cranberry-cereal bars, 148
  creamy cherry parfait, 131
  creamy vanilla frosting, 151
  crepes with creamy peach filling, 136–137
  frostings, 150, 151
  gingerbread, 142
  lemon poppy-seed cake, 141
  maple rice pudding, 132
  maple-soynut butter balls, 152
  mocha mousse, 133
  orange raisin balls, 147
  pecan pie, 129
  pumpkin cheesecake, 134
  pumpkin mousse, 134
  rhubarb cheese pie, 138
  rhubarb-strawberry custard pie, 128
  strawberry "ice cream," 144
  strawberry trifle, 135
diet, adding soyfoods to your, xvii–xviii
dips
  blue cheese, 47
  blue cheese & tofu spread, 3
  dill salmon spread, 5
  Louie dressing, 36, 74
  roasted bell pepper & tofu spread, 2
  roasted eggplant spread, 7
  southwestern hummus, 12
  tofu, 1
  tuna, 6
dressings
  avocado, 48
  blue cheese, 47
  buttermilk, 43
  creamy, 46
  Louie, 36, 74
  sesame, 39
drinks
  mango-banana smoothie, 126
  papaya-strawberry smoothie, 126

E

Edamame (green soybeans), xxiii, 41, 81
eggplant
  chicken & roasted vegetable pasta, 55
  roasted, spread, 7
  rollatina with marinara sauce, 58–59
eggs
  chile & ham puff, 119
  ham strata, 122
  southwestern scramble, 118
  soy bacon quiche, 123
estrogen, using soyfoods as alternative to,
  xii, xiii

F

feta cheese
  pasta & green soybean salad, 40–41
  vegetable-cheese filo slices, 10–11
fiber, list of soyfoods high in, xi
filo pastry
  onion-cheese strudel, 66–67
  vegetable-cheese filo slices, 10–11
flavonoids, x. *See also* phytochemicals
flax seed, 108
flour, soy, xxiv, xxv
  banana waffles, 112
  cherry-almond coffeecake, 114–115
  cornbread, 93
  cranberry-pumpkin muffins, 98
  cranberry scones, 101
  spiced fruit & nut yeast bread, 102–103
flour, white whole-wheat, 97
Food and Drug Administration (FDA), on soy
  protein, xv–xvi
French bread crisps, 5
frostings
  chocolate, 150
  creamy vanilla, 151

G

gas, passing, from overeating soybeans, xvii
Gimme Lean!™ (soy product), tomato pasta
  sauce, 54
ginger
  apricot & currant drop scones, 104
  banana bread, 100
  bread, 142
grits, soy, xxv, 117
  bulgur casserole, 86

ground beef
  beef & bean wraps, 65
  black bean, beef & tofu loaf, 62
  new-fashioned meat loaf, 63

H-I
ham
  ham strata, 122
  puff with egg and chile, 119
  schnitzel mit tofu, 69
health benefits of eating soyfoods, viii–xiv
  added fiber to diet, xi
  added source of protein, xv–xvi
  antioxidant, xi
  cancer, may prevent certain types of, xi–xii
  lowers cholesterol, x–xi, xv
  menopause, may help relieve symptoms of,
    xiii
  osteoporosis, may help prevent, xii–xiii
  reduces clot formation, xi
  reduces risk of heart disease, x–xi
heart disease, soyfoods may reduce risk of,
  x–xi
homocysteine, as risk factor for heart disease,
  xi
hummus, 12
isoflavones, viii–x. *See also* phytochemicals
  health benefits of, xii, xiii
  recommended daily intake, xiv
  soyfoods rich in, xii, xvi, xxix

L-M
lactose insufficient, soy milk for, xix
leeks, potato soup with, 19
lemon glaze, 96–97
lemon zest
  lemon poppy-seed cake, 141
  lemon poppy-seed muffins, 96–97
  rhubarb-strawberry custard pie, 128
  spiced fruit & nut yeast bread, 102–103
mail-order sources for soyfoods, 153
Main dishes
  bean quesadillas, 68
  beef & bean wraps, 65
  black bean, beef & tofu loaf, 62
  bulgur-vegetable burgers, 52–53
  chicken & roasted vegetable pasta, 55
  chicken & tempeh curry, 50
  chiles rellenos, 73

  dilled salmon patties, 74
  eggplant rollatina with marinara sauce,
    58–59
  meat loaf, new-fashioned, 63
  onion-cheese strudel, 66–67
  pecan & mushroom burgers, 51
  salmon crepes, 60–61
  schnitzel mit tofu, 69
  sloppy joes, 57
  stuffed bell peppers, 56
  taco noodle casserole, 72
  tempeh teriyaki, 75
  tomato-herb pasta sauce, 54
  tuna balls & mustard-chutney sauce,
    70–71
mango-banana smoothie, 126
maple syrup
  banana, 112–113
  maple-soynut butter balls, 152
  mocha mousse, 133
  rice pudding, 132
meat alternatives. *See* analogs
meat loaf
  black bean, beef & tofu loaf, 62
  new-fashioned, 63
menopause, soyfoods helping relieve
symptoms of, xiii
milk, soy. *See* soy milk
miso, xxiv
  barbecued tofu bites, 13
  black soybean soup, 25
  creamy broccoli soup, 24
  leek & potato soup, 19
  shrimp soup, 18
  vegetarian chili, 30
muffins. *See also* breads
  cranberry-pumpkin, 98
  double-corn, 92
  lemon poppy-seed, 96–97
  toasted pecan & currant, 95
mushrooms
  artichoke-stuffed, 4
  burgers, with toasted pecans, 51
  crimini & asparagus bake, 85

N-O
navy beans
  vegetarian chili, 30
  white bean & tofu salad, 32

nigari (soy-milk coagulating agent), xxix
organizations, 154
osteoporosis, soyfoods reduce risk of, xii–xiii

P-Q
pancakes
    blueberry, 106–107
    whole-wheat, 108–109
papaya
    avocado salad, 64
    strawberry smoothie, 126
pasta dishes
    chicken & roasted vegetables, 55
    chicken, baked tofu & noodle salad, 38
    green soybean salad, 40–41
    taco noodle casserole, 72
    tomato-herb pasta sauce, 54
peaches, creamy filling for crepes, 136–137
pecans
    pie, 129
    pumpkin mousse, 134
    toasted, cinnamon waffles, 110–111
    toasted, currant muffins, 95
    toasted, mushroom burgers, 51
phytates, xx
phytochemicals (plant chemicals), ix.
    See also flavonoids
phytoestrogens (plant estrogen), xiii
pies
    pastry crust, 129
    pecan, 129
    rhubarb-strawberry custard, 128
pine nuts, toasted, 87, 110
potatoes
    dilled potato salad, 33
    garlic & herb mashed, 83
    leek soup with, 19
    twice-baked, 88
prescription drugs, caution regarding using
    soyfoods instead of, xxi
prostate cancer, soyfoods may reduce risk of,
    xi, xii
protein
    digestion of, xx
    forms of, xxvii
    soyfoods containing, xv–xvi
pumpkin
    cheesecake,
    cranberry muffins, 98

curried soup, 16
    mousse, 134
quesadillas
    crab, 9
    stacked bean, 68

R
raisin orange balls, 147
rhubarb
    cheese pie, 138
    strawberry custard pie, 128
rice pudding with maple syrup, 132
roasted soybeans. *See* soynuts

S
Salads
    apple-cabbage slaw, 45
    chicken, baked tofu & noodle salad, 38
    crab Louie, 35
    curried tempeh & fruit salad, 44
    dilled potato salad, 33
    fried tofu with tossed greens, 42
    pasta & green soybean salad, 40–41
    tuna salad–stuffed tomatoes, 34
    two-bean & corn salad, 37
    white bean & tofu salad, 32
salmon
    chowder, 20–21
    crepes, 60–61
    dilled patties, 74
    dilled spread, 5
    smoked rolls, 8
salsa
    papaya-avocado, 64
    tomato-basil, 124–125
salt. *See* sodium
sauces
    avocado, 9
    jalapeño-flavored cheese, 89
    marinara, 58–59
    mustard-chutney, 70–71
    tomato-herb pasta, 54
sausages, pork, 121
scones
    apricot & currant drop, 104
    dried cranberry, 101
serum triglycerides, soyfoods lowers, x–xi
shoyu (soy sauce), xxvii
shrimp miso soup, 18

Side dishes
  bulgur casserole, 86
  cooked dried soybeans, 78–79
  couscous pilaf with green soybeans, 87
  creamed spinach casserole, 84
  easy spicy cheese sauce, 89
  garlic & herb mashed potatoes, 83
  green shelled soybeans, 80
  green soybeans, corn and tomatoes, 90
  green soybeans in pods, 81
  mushrooms & asparagus bake, 85
  rice and soybeans, 80
  roasted soynuts, 82
  twice-baked potatoes, 88
skin cancer, soyfoods may reduce risk of, xi,
  xii
smoothies
  mango-banana, 126
  papaya-strawberry, 126
sodium, soy products high in, xx
Soups
  black soybean soup, 25
  chicken–green chile stew, 17
  crab bisque, 26–27
  creamy broccoli soup, 24
  curried pumpkin soup, 16
  leek & potato soup, 19
  salmon chowder, 20–21
  shrimp miso soup, 18
  vegetable soup, 22–23
soy beverages. *See* soy milk
soy milk, xvii, xxv–xxvi
  fat content of, xvii
  for lactose insufficient, xix
  powdered form, using in, xxvi
  as protein source, xv
soy milk (recipes)
  apple bread, 99
  apricot & currant drop scones, 104
  banana waffles, 112
  blueberry coffeecake, 116
  blueberry pancakes, 106–107
  breakfast wraps, 120
  cherry-almond coffeecake, 114–115
  chocolate cookies, no-bake, 149
  chocolate frosting, 150
  chocolate granola bars, 146
  chocolate "ice cream," 145
  cornbread, 93

  crab bisque, 26–27
  cranberry-pumpkin muffins, 98
  cranberry scones, 101
  cream biscuits, 94
  creamed spinach casserole, 84
  creamy broccoli soup, 24
  crepes with creamy peach filling, 136–137
  curried pumpkin soup, 16
  leek & potato soup, 19
  Louie dressing, 36
  mushroom & asparagus bake, 85
  orange raisin balls, 147
  pecan & currant muffins, 95
  pecan-cinnamon waffles, 110
  rhubarb-strawberry custard pie, 128
  salmon chowder, 20–21
  salmon crepes, 60–61
  spiced fruit & nut yeast bread, 102–103
  spicy cheese sauce, 89
  strawberry "ice cream," 144
  taco noodle casserole, 72
  whole-wheat pancakes, 108–109
soy oil, xvi
soy powder, xxvii
  mango-banana smoothie, 126
  maple-soynut butter balls, 152
soy protein concentrates, xxvii
soy protein isolates, xxvii
soy sauces, xvi, xxvii, xx, 39
soybean oil, xxvi
soybeans
  black, xxii
  canned, xxiii
  dried, xxii
  eating raw, caution regarding, xx
  fiber, as source for, xi
  green, xxiii
  protein, as source for, xv
  slow cooker method, 79
  yellow, xxii
soybeans (recipes), 31
  beef & bean wraps, 65
  black bean, beef & tofu loaf, 62
  black bean chili, 28–29
  black soybean soup, 25
  chicken–green chile stew, 17
  couscous pilaf with green, 87
  dried, 78
  green, 80, 81

green, corn and tomatoes, 90
pasta & green soybean salad, 40–41
southwestern hummus, 12
stacked bean quesadillas, 68
two-bean & corn salad, 37
vegetable soup, 22–23
soyfoods
adding to diet, xvii–xviii
fat content of, xviii
health benefits of eating, viii–xiv
mail-order sources for, 153
organizations, 154
recommended daily intake, xiv
supplements, taking as, xviii–xix
using for substituting, xvii–xviii, xxiii
where to purchase, xvi
soynut butter, xxvi–xxvii, xviii
chocolate cookies, no-bake, 149
cranberry-cereal bars, 148
maple-soynut butter balls, 152
soynuts, xi
buttermilk dressing, 43
chicken, baked tofu & noodle salad, 38
chocolate granola bars, 146
maple-soynut butter balls, 152
roasted, 82
spinach, creamed casserole, 84
stews, chicken–green chile, 17
strawberries
"ice cream," 144
papaya smoothie, 126
rhubarb custard pie, 128
trifle, 135
strudel, onion-cheese, 66–67
substituting ingredients using soyfoods,
xvii–xviii, xxiii
beans, use green soybeans, xxiii
flour, use soy flour, 91
meat, use textured soy protein, xvii–xviii.
See also analogs
peanuts, use soynuts, xxvi
supermarkets, as source for soyfoods, xvi, xxii
sweet beans (shelled green soybeans), xxiii,
80
pasta & green soybean salad, 40–41
syrups. *See also* maple syrup
banana-maple, 112–113
double-apricot, 108–109
dried cherry, 110–111

orange-maple, 106–107

T
tamari (soy sauce), xxvii, 75. *See also*
soy sauces
tempeh, xi, xxvii, xxviii
chicken & tempeh curry, 50
curried tempeh & fruit salad, 44
egg, chile & ham puff, 119
roasted bell peppers, 56
roasted eggplant spread, 7
sloppy joes, 57
teriyaki, 75
vegetarian chili, 30
textured soy protein (TSP), xxvii, xxviii–xxix
black bean chili, 28–29
meat loaf, 63
meat substitute, xvii, xviii
pork sausages, 121
soups, 15
textured vegetable protein (TVP), xxviii–xxix
tofu, vii, viii, xv, xxix–xxx
freezing, xxx
how made, xxix
preparing, xxx
types of, vii, viii, xxix–xxx
regular, xxix
silken, xxix–xxx
tofu (recipes)
apple bread, 99
applesauce spice bars, 143
artichoke-stuffed mushrooms, 4
avocado sauce, 9
barbecued tofu bites, 13
black bean, beef & tofu loaf, 62
blue cheese & tofu spread, 3
blueberry coffeecake, 116
blueberry pancakes, 106–107
bulgur-vegetable burger, 52
carrot spice cake, 140
cherry-almond coffeecake, 114–115
cherry cheesecake, 131
chicken & roasted vegetable pasta, 55
chicken, baked tofu & noodle salad, 38
chiles rellenos, 73
chocolate brownies, 139
chocolate "ice cream," 145
corn muffins, 92
crab bisque, 26–27

creamed spinach casserole, 84
creamy broccoli soup, 24
creamy cherry parfait, 131
creamy dressing, 46
crepes with creamy peach filling, 136
curried pumpkin soup, 16
dilled salmon patties, 74
dip, 1
eggplant rollatina with marinara sauce, 58–59
fried, with tossed greens, 42
garlic & herbed mashed potatoes, 83
ginger banana bread, 100
gingerbread, 142
ham strata, 122
lemon poppy-seed cake, 141
maple rice pudding, 132
onion-cheese strudel, 66–67
papaya-strawberry smoothie, 126
pecan pie, 129
pumpkin cheesecake, 134
pumpkin mousse, 134
rhubarb cheese pie, 138
rhubarb-strawberry custard pie, 128
roasted bell pepper spread, 5
salmon crepes, 60–61
schnitzel mit tofu, 69
smoked salmon rolls, 8
southwestern egg scramble, 118
soy bacon quiche, 123
spicy tofu wrap, 42
stacked bean quesadillas, 68
strawberry "ice cream," 144
strawberry trifle, 135
toasted-pecan & mushroom burger, 51
toasted pecan–cinnamon waffles, 110–111
tuna balls, 70–71
tuna dip, 6
vegetable-cheese filo slices, 10–11
white bean & tofu salad, 32
zucchini frittata, 124
tomatoes
    basil salsa, 124–125
    green soybeans, corn and, 90
    herb pasta sauce, 54
    stuffed with tuna salad, 34
    two-bean & corn salad, 37
tortillas
    beef & bean wraps, 65
    breakfast wraps, 120
    stacked bean quesadillas, 68
    warming, 65
TSP. *See* textured soy protein
tuna
    balls with mustard-chutney sauce, 70
    dip, 6
    salad–stuffed tomatoes, 34
turkey, ground, in black bean chili, 28–29

V-W-Y-Z
veggie burgers
    bulgur-vegetable, 52–53
    toasted-pecan & mushroom burgers, 51
vitamin E, soyfoods containing, xi
waffles
    banana with banana-maple syrup, 112–113
    toasted pecan–cinnamon, 110–111
wraps
    beef & bean, 65
    breakfast, 120
    spicy tofu, 42
yogurt, soy, xxviii
    lemon poppy-seed muffins, 96
    pastry, 130
    twice-baked potatoes, 88
zucchini, frittata with tomato-basil salsa, 124–125